Responding to the AIDS Epidemic

Other books in the At Issue series:

At ✳ Issue

Responding to the AIDS Epidemic

Daniel A. Leone, *Book Editor*

Bonnie Szumski, *Publisher*
Helen Cothran, *Managing Editor*

GREENHAVEN PRESS
An imprint of Thomson Gale, a part of The Thomson Corporation

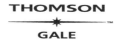

Detroit • New York • San Francisco • San Diego • New Haven, Conn.
Waterville, Maine • London • Munich

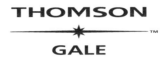

For more information, contact
Greenhaven Press
27500 Drake Rd.
Farmington Hills, MI 48331-3535
Or you can visit our Internet site at http://www.gale.com

Greenhaven Press anthologies primarily consist of previously published material taken from a variety of sources, including periodicals, books, scholarly journals, newspapers, government documents, and position papers from private and public organizations. These original sources are often edited for length and to ensure their accessibility for a young adult audience. The anthology editors also change the original titles of these works in order to clearly present the main thesis of each viewpoint and to explicitly indicate the opinion presented in the viewpoint. These alterations are made in consideration of both the reading and comprehension levels of a young adult audience. Every effort is made to ensure that Greenhaven Press accurately reflects the original intent of the authors included in this anthology.

LIBRARY OF CONGRESS CATALOGING-IN-PUBLICATION DATA
Responding to the AIDS epidemic / Daniel A. Leone, book editor.

Responding to the AIDS epidemic / Daniel A. Leone, book editor.
    p. cm. — (At issue)
Includes bibliographical references and index.
ISBN 0-7377-2745-4 (lib. bdg. : alk. paper) —
ISBN 0-7377-2746-2 (pbk. : alk. paper)
    1. AIDS (Disease)—Cross-cultural studies. 2. AIDS (Disease)—Prevention.
3. AIDS (Disease)—Government policy—United States. I. Leone, Daniel A.,
1969– . II. At issue (San Diego, Calif.)
RA643.8.R47 2006
614.5'99392—dc22   2005052691

Printed in the United States of America

Contents

Introduction

In 1981 the Centers for Disease Control announced that it had identified a new disease that attacked the immune system. Almost twenty-five years later, the disease, Acquired Immune Deficiency Syndrome (AIDS), has spread across the globe, killing millions. According to UNAIDS, a United Nations organization that tracks the global spread of AIDS, the epidemic has claimed over 20 million lives. UNAIDS estimates that nearly 40 million more are infected with HIV, the human immunodeficiency virus that causes AIDS. Among those aged 15–59, AIDS is the leading cause of death worldwide.

AIDS cases have been reported in all parts of the world, but most appear in poor, developing countries. In 2004 alone, 4.9 million people worldwide became infected with HIV. Over 80 percent of these new cases came from sub-Saharan Africa and Southeast Asia. East Asia and Latin America were the next hardest hit, with 290,000 and 240,000 new cases, respectively. In contrast, North America and Western Europe had 44,000 and 21,000 new cases, respectively. Sub-Saharan Africa is by far the world region most affected by HIV/AIDS. Over 25 million infected people, 64 percent of global HIV/AIDS cases, live in this region. The incidence among adults has reached an epidemic proportion of 7.4 percent. South Africa has the highest adult HIV/AIDS rate of any country in the world, with an estimated 21.4 percent of its adult population having become infected. This stands in startling contrast to the global average of adult HIV/AIDS prevalence, which is 1.1 percent. Even more dramatic is the contrast to adult rates in wealthy regions of the world such as North America and western Europe. In these regions the average adult incidence rate is below one-half of a percent.

Experts have developed several theories to explain why the disease flourishes in the developing regions of the world. Some analysts argue that undeveloped economies and poverty are the primary reasons AIDS has spread so dramatically in the developing world. They maintain, for example, that poor countries do not have the resources to fund a sufficient quantity of drug treatments to control the spread of the disease in a population so disproportionately infected. According to Peter Piot, the executive director of UNAIDS, "Last year, 30,000 people in sub-Saharan Africa received antiretroviral drugs; in the same period, 2.2 million people died of AIDS." These commentators also claim that risky behaviors that spread HIV are more prevalent in poverty-stricken countries. Starving women, for example, sometimes resort to prostitution to earn money for food and basic needs. Unfortunately, these analysts assert, in an effort to escape starvation, these women not only expose themselves to HIV infection but also further spread the disease.

Some experts argue that poverty alone cannot explain widespread AIDS infection rates in the developing world. These commentators claim that the leaders of many developing nations are uninformed about AIDS and therefore fail to take action strong enough to combat the spread of the disease. For example, South African president Thabo Mbeki, they assert, is not convinced that HIV causes AIDS and therefore does not allow AIDS patients to be treated with antiviral drugs that prevent the disease from spreading. Ben Barber, State Department correspondent for the *Washington Times,* states, "Mbeki's refusal to let antiretroviral drugs be administered to AIDS patients has allowed HIV to be transmitted unchecked." Mbeki's lack of political leadership, his failure to mobilize public support and rally against the disease, explains why South Africa has the highest AIDS prevalence of any country in the world, these analysts maintain.

Some researchers contend that ineffective public health systems better explain AIDS prevalence in developing nations. A series of studies published in 2003 by the *International Journal of STD & AIDS* suggests that "medical transmission" has spread AIDS in Africa. The studies imply that clinics funded and approved by the United Nations are spreading the disease with infected needles, blood, and medical instruments. These analysts point to the disproportionate number of women stricken with AIDS in the developing world to support their theory. They argue that many Western-funded clinics in Africa are designed to promote birth control and sterilization. According to experts, women receiving treatments to prevent them from bearing children are accidentally infected with HIV-infected needles and instruments. Steven Mosher of the Population Research Institute explains: "Women and girls account for such a high percentage of HIV/AIDS victims in Africa because they are infected during procedures designed to disable their reproductive systems." Mosher suggests that these UN-endorsed clinics, which are promoted as a cure for AIDS, are actually causing the spread of the disease.

Still another theory explaining the prevalence of AIDS in the developing world postulates that the AIDS virus itself differs in the developed and developing world. Harvard professor Max Essex discovered five strains of HIV in different parts of the world and labeled them A, B, C, D, and E. Essex found that all strains except the B strain can be easily transmitted through heterosexual intercourse. While the B strain does not easily transmit through heterosexual intercourse, it does transmit effectively through homosexual intercourse. The B strain is found predominately in the developed countries of North America and western Europe, where AIDS has spread more readily among the homosexual population. Essex argues that infection rates in the developed world have been relatively low because the HIV strain found in these regions has not as readily spread to the larger heterosexual population. Furthermore, he suggests that unless developed nations combat AIDS more aggressively worldwide, the HIV strains that spread through heterosexual intercourse will eventually spread to developed countries, creating an explosion of infection rates in these regions as well. Essex maintains, "If we are not motivated by the ethical mandate of protecting millions of people at risk in developing countries, perhaps the threat of newer and even deadlier HIV epidemics at home will goad us to action."

Experts continue to debate which of these theories best explains the disproportionate spread of AIDS in developing nations. Since the response to the AIDS epidemic in the developing and developed world is in many ways determined by its perceived causes, the policies that will best respond to the epidemic are equally contentious. The authors in *At Issue: Responding to the AIDS Epidemic* debate which response strategies will be most effective in controlling the global spread of AIDS.

1

The Global AIDS Epidemic Is a Serious Problem

Ed Susman

Ed Susman is a freelance writer and a regular contributor to United Press International.

As of March 2004, 20 million people worldwide have died of AIDS and 40 million have been infected. Africa has the highest prevalence of the disease; in fact, AIDS is the leading cause of death on the continent. Over fifteen nations in Africa have HIV infection rates exceeding 10 percent of the population. In Asia, AIDS infection rates are growing rapidly, particularly in China and India, the two most populated nations in the world. AIDS cases are also mounting in the Caribbean, Latin America, and eastern Europe. While western Europe and the United States have relatively low rates of infection compared to the rest of the world, AIDS continues to spread among homosexuals, bisexuals, and injecting drug users in these regions.

Sometime early in the twentieth century, possibly preceding the Great Depression, a virus carried by African primates jumped from one species to another, becoming HIV (human immunodeficiency virus). Fifty years later, on continents far from sub-Saharan Africa, HIV was discovered and identified as the cause of AIDS (autoimmune deficiency syndrome).

The AIDS epidemic has become a mounting global tragedy,

with 20 million killed and 40 million infected. Worldwide in 2003, according to estimates from the Joint United Nations Programme on HIV/AIDS (UNAIDS), roughly five million people were infected with HIV. More than three million [were] expected to die from complications of the disease in 2004.

In Africa, the pandemic's effects are unmatched in their severity and tragic consequences. About 29.6 million of those infected with or dying of HIV/AIDS live in sub-Saharan Africa, where the virus spread to 3.2 million more people in 2003 alone and 58 percent of those living with HIV are women. Although the horror and extent of the disease on the African continent have brought promises of assistance from world leaders, including President George W. Bush, a combination of poverty, government inaction, myth, and stigma continues to drive the epidemic to levels that are difficult for citizens of the developed countries to comprehend.

Highly opportunistic and robust, HIV thrives and spreads among humans primarily because of promiscuous sexual behavior, unsafe medical injections, needle sharing among users of addictive drugs, mother to child transmission, and, in some parts of the world, tainted blood products. For this article, however, the focus is not on the behaviors but on the national-level consequences and responses in six regions of the world: Africa, Asia, the Caribbean and Latin America, eastern Europe, western Europe, and the United States.

Africa

In Africa, where 16 nations have disease prevalence rates that exceed 10 percent—20 times the 0.5 percent HIV incidence rate in the United States and western Europe—many governments have ignored the epidemic that fills hospital wards and leaves millions of homeless orphans in its wake.

Nearly five million South Africans—15 percent of the population—are infected with HIV. Nevertheless, the government has for more than three years blocked efforts to provide pregnant women with drugs that can prevent transmission of HIV to their babies. It now promises that treatment programs will be in place by 2005.

It is estimated that 8,000 babies are born to HIV-infected mothers each month in South Africa. Without treatment, 33 to 40 percent of those infants will have HIV. With treatment, less than 2 percent would be born with HIV, which kills most infected babies before they are four years old.

An estimated 600 people die from AIDS every day in South Africa, and thousands more die in Botswana, Swaziland, Zimbabwe, Malawi, and all across Africa. Only in a few places are drugs being distributed; only in a few countries are preventive messages being heeded.

Though these numbers are grim, the human impact behind them is numbing. As Dr. Thomas Quinn, professor of medicine at Johns Hopkins University in Baltimore, explained: "One has to consider Africa's main agricultural society. Seven million farmers have died due to AIDS. One has to ask who is farming the land.

> *The AIDS epidemic has become a mounting global tragedy.*

"There is also the educational process as well as the working process," he said. "Eighty-five percent of teacher deaths in the last 20 years have been due to AIDS.

"In fact, AIDS is the leading cause of death within the continent. Because it affects many people in their young, reproductive ages, we are left with a very large number of orphans. These children are not necessarily infected with HIV but are left behind due to the premature death of their parents.

"From the global perspective, the HIV epidemic has reversed many of the developmental gains that have been achieved in many areas of the world, particularly those made over the last three decades," said Quinn. "There has been an economic decline, particularly on the African continent, with estimates of that decline ranging from 10 to 40 percent—a staggering figure in an area that is already economically fragile.

"One result is health-system chaos. In some places, 50 to 70 or 80 percent of hospital beds may be occupied by HIV-infected people with opportunistic infections, many of which go untreated. All of this results in a spiraling factor of political instability," Quinn noted.

"Africa is where AIDS has entrenched itself in the last two to three decades and is still spiraling out of control. The spread of HIV continues relentlessly across the continent."

On a more positive note, he observed that some countries

are making a difference in limiting its spread and in treating HIV-infected patients. Uganda, for example, has successfully reduced the incidence and prevalence of HIV through behavioral education programs, and Botswana and Senegal are implementing effective treatment programs.

Asia

While Africa's social, economic, and humanitarian catastrophe has caught the world's attention, a pending AIDS disaster in Asia barely causes a blip on the radar screen.

Officials are aware of the disease's growing incidence in India and China, which are home to more than 2 billion people. They have sounded alarms, but in vulnerable, undereducated, and poverty-stricken areas, those warnings may go unheard.

Consider India. Officially, just under 4 million people are living with HIV infection in the world's most populous democracy, but many doctors in the field think this figure is underestimated.

UNAIDS reports some progress: "New behavioral studies in India suggest that prevention efforts directed at specific populations such as female sex workers and injecting drug users are paying dividends in some states, in the form of higher HIV/AIDS knowledge and condom use.

> *'Africa is where AIDS has entrenched itself in the last two to three decades.'*

"However," it reports, "HIV prevalence among those key groups continues to increase in some states, underlining the need for well-planned and sustained interventions on a large scale."

In neighboring Bangladesh, a nation the size of Wisconsin but with a population of 140 million, officially only a few hundred people have HIV infection, said Dr. A.Q.M. Serajul Islam, professor of dermatology and sexually transmitted diseases at Chittagong Medical College and Hospital.

"We screened 400 men at our clinic," he said, "and two of those men were positive for HIV." While that would indicate an infection rate of 0.5 percent at the clinic, Islam was more disturbed by the reactions of his patients.

"They are both married," he said, "but neither of them wanted to have his wife tested. Neither of them even wanted his wife to know that he had HIV." He said that women in Bangladesh seldom receive standard health care and rarely would receive testing for any sexually transmitted disease, let alone AIDS.

In China, which has a population of 1.3 billion, HIV infection is spreading rapidly—especially among injecting drug users. Infected blood products also are contributing to the spread of the disease there.

"The epidemic in China shows no signs of abating," the UNAIDS report stated. "Official estimates put the number of people living with HIV in China at 1 million in mid-2002. Unless effective responses rapidly take hold, a total of 10 million Chinese will have acquired HIV by the end of the decade." To put it another way, 10 million people is equivalent to the entire population of Belgium.

The Caribbean and Latin America

Although AIDS was recognized and identified in the United States and Europe in the 1980s, the extent of the disease throughout the Caribbean and Latin America is still underappreciated. According to UNAIDS: "In several Caribbean countries, adult HIV prevalence rates are surpassed only by the rates experienced in sub-Saharan Africa—making this the second-most affected region in the world."

"I don't think that the situation in Latin America and the Caribbean will ever come close to Africa, where infection rates among adults exceed 10, 15, or 20 percent. But there are already a number of countries in Latin America that have infection rates that exceed 1 percent—and that really is troublesome," said Dr. Richard Keenlyside of the Centers for Disease Control and Prevention in Atlanta.

Reports show that the HIV infection rate is higher than 1 percent in 12 countries in the region. This might not seem very high, but at that level the disease already affects overall life expectancy and economic development.

Among the nations that have prevalence rates above 1 percent are impoverished Haiti at 6 percent and the Bahamas at 3.5 percent. Throughout the region, 1.9 million people—nearly half a million in the Caribbean—are infected with HIV.

"We are also concerned about the rising epidemic in Guyana," said Keenlyside. The small nation on South America's Caribbean shore has an HIV prevalence rate of 2.7 percent among adults between the ages of 15 and 49.

Keenlyside, associate director for external relations and public health practice for the CDC's Global AIDS Program, said he is encouraged by work being done in the Bahamas, Barbados, and Brazil.

A regional anomaly is Cuba, with an AIDS prevalence rate only one-tenth that of the United States. Cuba controls HIV spread with compulsory HIV education, generic antiretroviral drugs, and universal, mandatory testing, but Keenlyside doubts that such strict methods could be copied in democratic nations.

Eastern Europe

As knowledge of how to control the AIDS epidemic improves, hopes are raised that its spread will be checked. Eastern Europe is one place where those hopes are illusory, as there is a great chasm between knowledge and the political will to act.

Dr. Scott Hammer, professor of infectious diseases at Columbia University, bit his lip and thought about how to describe the AIDS epidemic in eastern Europe. "Explosive," he said. "Explosive."

In countries such as Belarus, Ukraine, Russia, and Uzbekistan, the epidemic is roaring through populations of injecting drug users and is evident among people with other sexually transmitted diseases. In the region, 1.2 million people are infected with HIV.

> *In China, which has a population of 1.3 billion, HIV infection is spreading rapidly.*

The 28 states that make up eastern Europe are strapped for cash to run prevention campaigns and treatment programs. More tragically, the governments of the region have generally avoided learning anything from the mistakes made in the West and Africa, where the epidemic is more mature. Dr. Peter Piot, executive director of UNAIDS, singled out Russia for specific criticism, saying the nation expends few resources in fighting the epidemic and does not even have a high-ranking official in charge of those meager efforts.

That is in light of shocking epidemics such as the one in industrial Togliatti, a city with a population of about 750,000, located on the Volga River about 700 miles south of Moscow. Among injecting drug users in that city, about 56 percent were HIV infected, said Ali Judd, a researcher at the Imperial College Faculty of Medicine in London. The year before, 41 percent of those subjects had been HIV negative. More ominous, 43 percent of the drug users surveyed were sex workers.

> **"The AIDS epidemic in the United States is far from over."**

"We know from past experience," said Hammer, "that once HIV is in the injecting drug population and among sex workers, the virus most likely is already widespread." Outbreaks such as the one in Togliatti are occurring throughout the region, said Dr. Alex Wodak, director of the alcohol and drug treatment service at St. Vincent's Hospital, Sydney, Australia.

Western Europe

While the situation in eastern Europe is worrisome, the wealthier states of western Europe have their own problems with the epidemic. Up to 10 percent of people infected with HIV have a mutated virus that is resistant to at least one class of drugs used to treat the disease.

"Transmission of resistant virus occurs," said Dr. David van de Vijver, an epidemiologist at the University Medical Center in Utrecht, the Netherlands. The pan-European survey looked at rates of drug-resistant virus from 17 countries. In western Europe, an estimated 570,000 people are living with HIV/AIDS.

While most of those countries have stable rates of overall infection, there are still pockets of alarming increases in new infection rates, notably in cities in Portugal and Italy. "We were used to thinking that the epidemic in western Europe was stable," said Lucas Wiessing, a researcher with the European Monitoring Centre for Drugs and Drug Addiction in Lisbon. "But we have found that despite prevention measures, HIV transmission continues at high rates among sub-groups of injecting drug users in some countries."

"The situation in Portugal is very scary," said van de Vijver.

The United States

Even in the United States, government agencies are expressing concerns that the "stable" epidemic is showing signs of instability. In this country, 900,000 people are infected with HIV; 180,000 of these are women, 10,000 are children under the age of 15, and there are hints that infection rates are on the rise again. According to Dr. Harold Jaffe, director of the CDC's National Center for HIV, Sexually Transmitted Disease, and Tuberculosis, an increasing number of new HIV infections are being diagnosed among gay and bisexual men. From 2001 to 2002, the number of new HIV diagnoses per year rose 7.1 percent among that population; in the three years from 1999 to 2002, the number of new HIV diagnoses per year has increased by 17.7 percent.

"The AIDS epidemic in the United States is far from over," said Jaffe. "While effective treatments are crucial in our fight against HIV, preventing infection in the first place is still the only true protection against the serious and fatal consequences of this disease."

Undoubtedly, a few rays of sunshine may pierce the darkness of the HIV/AIDS pandemic, especially in the wealthier nations. For the majority of the 40 million people now infected, however—and the millions more who will become infected with the killer disease this year and next—the sunshine eludes them. Instead, the shadow of a disease that robs people of their most productive years and extends over families, communities, and nations spreads relentlessly across the landscape.

2

The African AIDS Epidemic Is Exaggerated

Tom Bethell

Tom Bethell is a senior editor of The American Spectator, *a conservative news magazine.*

The prevalence of AIDS in Africa has been exaggerated. While the World Health Organization has confirmed slightly over a million AIDS cases in Africa, the media reports the number infected to be over 30 million. However, media estimates are based on a relaxed definition of AIDS used in African nations. Because of their high costs, HIV tests are not always given in Africa. The AIDS diagnosis is therefore often based on symptoms alone. If a patient exhibits the major symptoms of AIDS—such as 10 percent weight loss, prolonged diarrhea, and a persistent cough—they are diagnosed with AIDS. However, many diseases such as malaria commonly found on the continent have the same symptoms and are being inaccurately diagnosed as AIDS.

Anthony Fauci has directed the Institute for Allergy and Infectious Diseases [NIAID] almost since AIDS began. It is a part of the Hydra-headed thing called the National Institutes for Health. I bumped into him not long ago at a Starbucks in Washington, D.C. It was a Saturday morning and he was wearing a shiny black jacket, but he was easily recognizable from his frequent television appearances. He told me he had spent his entire career at NIAID. Since AIDS hit the headlines his agency's budget has soared, and he deserves no little credit for that.

I told him I had heard that in Africa you don't need an HIV test to be diagnosed with AIDS. "They don't do it because the test is so expensive," Fauci said. He added that when HIV testing is done (e.g. on pregnant women in pre-natal clinics in South Africa) the estimated HIV-infection rate is confirmed. Diagnosis without a test is done "more for economic reasons than anything else," he said.

A Broader Definition

It's important to remember that AIDS is defined as about 25 pre-existing diseases in conjunction with a "positive" test for antibodies to the human immunodeficiency virus. They don't test for the virus itself. They test for antibodies to it. But in sub-Saharan Africa, they don't have to do the test! Think about that. If you see a doctor, and you have certain symptoms, the authorities can count you as an "HIV-AIDS" case. What are the major symptoms? Fever for a month; weight loss of ten percent; and prolonged diarrhea. A persistent cough is another.

What this means is that traditional African diseases, common in areas with a tropical climate, open latrines and contaminated water, are now called something else: AIDS.

> **" In Africa you don't need an HIV test to be diagnosed with AIDS. "**

This key relaxation of what "AIDS" means in Africa was worked out at a 1985 conference in Bangui, in the Central African Republic. The conference was organized by the U.S. Centers for Disease Control [CDC]. The "Bangui definition" of African AIDS was duly reported in *Science* and in one or two medical journals, but it has not yet been reported by our major newspapers. The principal culprit has been Lawrence K. Altman of the *New York Times*. He is himself a former public health officer and worked for the CDC before joining the *Times*. Like Fauci, he has been a major player in the AIDS story from the beginning. He wrote the first AIDS article, in 1981. And he is still on the case. He was actually at Bangui for the 1985 conference. He wrote a big story for the *Times*, filling an entire inside page, with a "box" on the Bangui meeting. But it merely reported on a new "hospital surveillance system to determine the extent of AIDS." Dr. Altman failed to disclose that AIDS could now be diagnosed without an HIV test, and he hasn't mentioned it since.

It's worth noting that Mark Schoof, a *Village Voice* reporter (since hired by the *Wall Street Journal*), spent months in Africa in 1999 working on AIDS and won the Pulitzer Prize for his series. While in Africa he contracted malaria. As a result, he could be counted as an AIDS case by the Bangui definition.

HIV Tests May Indicate Other Conditions

Dr. Fauci had said that when HIV tests are conducted in Africa, they confirm the Bangui-based estimates. But the problem is that HIV tests react to lots of other conditions in addition to HIV. "They do not specifically identify HIV antibodies," says Christine Maggiore. She is the director of Alive & Well AIDS Alternatives, based in Los Angeles. Some years ago, although healthy, she was misleadingly diagnosed as "HIV positive." She provides the following rebuttal: "The antibody tests detect certain proteins that are not unique or specific to HIV antibodies and that may correspond to antibodies produced in response to over 60 conditions including colds, flu, immunizations, herpes, hepatitis, blood transfusions, parasites, TB, malaria and even pregnancy."

The conditions that produce false positives are abundant in African countries. Most Africans lack access to safe drinking water, over 60 percent have no sanitation. Human and animal excrement find their way into the water supply. In South Africa, where conditions are above African average, poor people may be reduced to scooping up drinking water from puddles. Yet AIDS, Inc. is confident that what Africans who meet the Bangui criteria more than anything need is the latest high-tech drugs such as protease inhibitors.

AIDS Drug Dangers

Worse, the AIDS establishment has suppressed a decade of mounting evidence about just how dangerous these drugs are. South Africa's President Thabo Mbeki has been under tremendous pressure to administer nevirapine to the babies of women found to be "HIV positive" when pregnant. The drug causes liver failure; a U.S. health-care worker with a needle-stick accident required a liver transplant after taking nevirapine. D. David Steele, an attorney in the Bay Area, recently filed a lawsuit on behalf of a plaintiff who was routinely treated with the drug after puncturing his finger with a stray needle. First developed as cancer chemotherapy, the suit claims that doctors failed to warn of AZT's potential toxic effects.

> **// The conditions that produce false positives [in HIV tests] are abundant in African countries. //**

Recently I interviewed Dr. David Rasnick, also in the Bay Area. A biochemist who holds patents on protease-type drugs, he is a member of Mbeki's AIDS Advisory Panel. The drugs used to treat AIDS patients are hazardous, he said. "Liver failure is the primary cause of death for American and European AIDS patients [who obediently take the drugs], even though liver disease is not one of the AIDS defining diseases." He pointed out that NIH has now abandoned its earlier recommendation that HIV positive patients be "hit early, hit hard." (That idea was pushed by AIDS researcher David Ho, *Time*'s 1996 "Man of the Year.")

An Exaggerated Number of AIDS Cases

What about the "pandemic" that is "ravaging Africa," at least in the headlines? Rasnick said: "In the past twenty years, the population of sub-Saharan Africa has increased by 274 million people, almost equal to the population of the United States." The World Health Organization's cumulative total of clinically confirmed AIDS cases in Africa through 2001 is 1.09 million. The far higher numbers routinely bandied about are simply guesses generated by the Bangui definition and validated by gullible journalists pushing photographs of thin men lying on cots. A *Rolling Stone* investigation could find no evidence of excess deaths in South Africa. What about the "20 million orphans" we read about? If one parent is dead or "missing" then their children can be called "orphans." The whole thing is a crock.

A recent discussion with an aide to a U.S. senator shed some light on what is really going on. Of course, big money is involved—$15 billion over the next five years from U.S. taxpayers. But there's something else. It always has been a major embarrassment that AIDS is predominantly male. Real infectious diseases aren't supposed to work that way. To avoid having to label it a "gay disease," a new slogan was confected: "We are all at risk."

The fact is that heterosexual transmission of the virus is almost impossible. Nancy Padian's study of 450 heterosexual couples with one infected partner showed no new infections after ten years. But then along comes African AIDS with its convenient local definition—and seeming evidence that AIDS is evenly divided between the sexes. We'll leave aside that this hypothesis imputes gross promiscuity to Africans. Senator Jeff Sessions of Alabama held hearings on the greater likelihood that HIV in Africa is transmitted by dirty needles in rundown hospitals and clinics. But Senator Kennedy was indignant that these hearings were held at all. Why? He does the bidding of the gay lobby. Heterosexual transmission is politically imperative to them.

3

Promoting Sexual Abstinence Will Reduce the Spread of AIDS

Rich Lowry

Rich Lowry is an editor of the conservative National Review.

Promoting sexual abstinence and marital fidelity has proven to reduce HIV rates. In the mid-1980s the president of Uganda, concerned about the threat of AIDS in his country, began a prevention program that aggressively promoted these practices. Researchers who followed the program report that increases in marital fidelity and decreases in sexual activity led to a decline in HIV cases. Despite the program's success, AIDS activists refuse to promote these prevention strategies because they feel that asking people to stop having sex is a human-rights violation. Failing to promote a proven AIDS-fighting strategy that will reduce the spread of AIDS and save lives is unconscionable.

World AIDS Day came and went with barely any notice of the fact that a kind of vaccine against HIV has been researched, tested and is available to save countless lives in Africa.

It was first developed during the late 1980s in Uganda, where it has created the biggest drop in HIV prevalence in the world. It hasn't yet been patented or advertised, but it has a name: abstinence and marital fidelity.

According to a U.S. Agency for International Development [USAID] study, in Uganda "national HIV prevalence peaked at around 15 percent in 1991, and had fallen to five percent as of 2001. This dramatic decline in prevalence is unique worldwide."

In the mid-1980s, when it became clear that AIDS was on the rise in Uganda, President Yoweri Museveni adopted a program that, as Arthur Allen has written in the *New Republic*, "would become known as ABC, for Abstain, Be faithful or wear a Condom—very much in order of emphasis."

> **"** *The effect [of promoting abstinence and marital fidelity] on HIV rates has been nearly miraculous.* **"**

Museveni essentially led a crusade against having sex outside of marriage. You can almost hear the clucking of "progressives" in the West: How quaint. How prudish. How unrealistic.

Try, instead: How wondrously effective.

The Success of Abstinence in Uganda

According to a study of one Ugandan district, almost 60 percent of youths age 13-16 reported engaging in sexual activity in 1994, but by 2001, the number had plummeted to less than 5 percent. The USAID study reports that compared with men in other sub-Saharan African countries, Uganda males are "less likely to have ever had sex (in the 15-19-year-old range), more likely to be married and keep sex within marriage, and less likely to have multiple partners."

The effect on HIV rates has been nearly miraculous. Researcher Rand Stoneburner estimates that Uganda's approach has been almost as effective as an HIV vaccine.

So, where's the shouting from the rooftops?

The silence about Uganda has to do with the fact that the condom, that sacred totem of the AIDS establishment, didn't initially play much of a role in ABC's success. As late as 1995—by which time HIV was already firmly on the decline—only 16 percent in Ugandan males reported ever using one.

In contrast, as Allen reports, Botswana and Zimbabwe, the two countries in the world with the highest rates of HIV prevalence, are both relatively condom-friendly. In a 1999 study, more than 70 percent of Zimbabwean males reported using a condom in their most recent high-risk sex act.

AIDS activists aren't picketing international organizations, demanding that they spread the Uganda model, because they have a blind spot. For them, urging people not to have sex almost constitutes a human-rights violation.

The researchers who have simply followed the Uganda data to its logical conclusion find themselves isolated in the AIDS world. "A lot of my colleagues get very wary at the sound of language urging behavioral changes," says one lonely expert, Harvard researcher Edward C. Green. "It sounds judgmental, moralistic. But it's hard to argue with success."

Abstinence Is Resisted by Many AIDS Activists

Difficult or not—there is still an ongoing effort to argue with success. The *Washington Post* . . . reported on "the war" on AIDS in Botswana: "Bill Gates is bankrolling the assault. A top pharmaceutical firm is supplying ammunition. And Harvard University researchers are developing new weapons."

Given the devastation in Botswana, where life expectancy is down from age 65 to less than 40, it is understandable to want to "try anything." But it's unforgivable not to try what has proven to work. Money, pills and experts all might help, but are besides the point absent a new ethic of sexual responsibility.

Now, Uganda shouldn't be mistaken for a chapter of the Christian Coalition. Condom use among high-risk groups has consolidated Uganda's gains, and social acceptance of HIV-positive people is quite high. But the AIDS establishment will never act on Uganda's central lesson until it gives up its total devotion to the idea of judgment-free sexual self-expression.

In the meantime, Africa dies.

4

Promoting Condom Use Will Reduce the Spread of AIDS

World Health Organization et al.

The World Health Organization, Joint United Nations Programme on HIV/AIDS, and the United Nations Population Fund are international health organizations dedicated to controlling and eliminating the spread of AIDS worldwide.

Condoms are the most effective tool available to reduce the spread of AIDS. Research shows that condom use reduces the transmission of HIV among heterosexual couples. To be most effective, AIDS prevention programs should make low-cost condoms widely available and work to overcome gender and cultural factors that reduce their usage. In many societies, men are opposed to the use of condoms and women lack the power to mandate their use. Both men and women should be encouraged to use condoms and should have equal access to them.

Prevention is the mainstay of the response to AIDS. Condoms are an integral and essential part of comprehensive prevention and care programmes, and their promotion must be accelerated. The AIDS epidemic is not levelling off. In 2003, an estimated 4.8 million people became newly infected with HIV—more than in any previous year. About 50% of them were young people 15 to 24 years old, with young girls at greater risk of infection than boys.

World Health Organization, Joint United Nations Program on HIV/AIDS, and United Nations Population Fund, "Position Statement on Condoms and HIV Prevention," www.who.int, July 2004. Copyright © 2004 by the World Health Organization. Reproduced by permission.

The Condom Is Very Effective Against AIDS

The male latex condom is the single, most efficient, available technology to reduce the sexual transmission of HIV and other sexually transmitted infections. The search for new preventive technologies such as HIV vaccines and microbicides continues to make progress, but condoms will remain the key preventive tool for many, many years to come. Condoms are a key component of combination prevention strategies individuals can choose at different times in their lives to reduce their risks of sexual exposure to HIV. These include delay of sexual initiation, abstinence, being safer by being faithful to one's partner when both partners are uninfected and consistently faithful, reducing the number of sexual partners, and correct and consistent use of condoms.

Conclusive evidence from extensive research among heterosexual couples in which one partner is infected with HIV shows that correct and consistent condom use significantly reduces the risk of HIV transmission from both men to women, and also from women to men. Laboratory studies show that male latex condoms are impermeable to infectious agents contained in genital secretions. To ensure safety and efficacy, condoms must be manufactured to the highest international standards. They must be procured according to the quality assurance procedures established by the WHO [World Health Organization], UNFPA [United Nations Fund for Population Activities] and UNAIDS [Joint United Nations Programme on HIV/AIDS] and they should be stored away from direct heat sources. Prevention programmes need to ensure that high-quality condoms are accessible to those who need them, when they need them, and that people have the knowledge and skills to use them correctly.

Universal Access to Condoms Is Crucial

Condoms must be readily available universally, either free or at low cost, and promoted in ways that help overcome social and personal obstacles to their use. Condom use is more likely when people can access them at no cost or at greatly subsidized prices. Effective condom promotion targets not only the general population, but also people at higher risk of HIV exposure, especially women, young people, sex workers and their clients, injecting drug users and men who have sex with men. UNFPA estimates that the [recent] supply of condoms in low- and middle-income countries falls 40% short of the number required (the condom 'gap'). Despite the gap, international funding for condom procurement has declined. . . . Collective actions at all levels are needed to support efforts of countries, especially those that depend on external assistance, in condom procurement, promotion and distribution.

> *The male latex condom is the single, most efficient, available technology to reduce the sexual transmission of HIV.*

HIV prevention education and condom promotion must overcome the challenges of complex gender and cultural factors. Young girls and women are regularly and repeatedly denied information about, and access to, condoms. Often they do not have the power to negotiate the use of condoms. In many social contexts, men are resistant to the use of condoms. This needs to be recognized in designing condom promotion programmes. Female condoms can provide women with more control in protecting themselves. However, women will remain highly vulnerable to HIV exposure, until men and women share equal decision-making powers in their interpersonal relationships.

Condom Use Has Been Effective in Many Countries

Condoms have played a decisive role in HIV prevention efforts in many countries. Condoms have helped to reduce HIV infection rates where AIDS has already taken hold and curtailed the broader spread of HIV in settings where the epidemic is still concentrated in specific populations. Condoms have also encouraged safer sexual behaviour more generally. Recent analysis of the AIDS epidemic in Uganda has confirmed that increased condom use, in conjunction with delay in age of first sexual intercourse and reduction of sexual partners, was an important factor in the decline of HIV prevalence in the 1990s. Thailand's efforts to de-stigmatize condoms and its targeted condom promotion for sex workers and their clients dramatically reduced HIV infections in these populations and helped reduce the spread of the epidemic to the general population. A similar policy in Cambodia has helped stabilize national prevalence, while substantially decreasing prevalence among sex workers. In addition, Brazil's early and vigorous condom promotion among the general population and vulnerable groups has successfully contributed to sustained control of the epidemic.

Increased access to antiretroviral treatment creates the need and the opportunity for accelerated condom promotion. The success of antiretroviral therapy in industrialized countries in reducing illness and prolonging life can alter the perception of risk associated with HIV. A perception of low-risk and a sense of complacency can lead to unprotected sex through reduced or non-consistent condom use. Promotion of correct and consistent condom use within antiretroviral treatment programmes, and within reproductive health and family planning services, is essential to reduce further opportunities for HIV transmission. Rapid scale-up of voluntary HIV testing accompanied by counselling is needed to meet the prevention needs of all people, whether they are HIV-positive or negative.

5

AIDS Medications Must Be Made Widely Available

Gary Karch

Gary Karch, an environmental activist, serves as media director for the Michigan Positive Action Coalition, an advocacy group for people living with AIDS.

AIDS medications must be made readily available worldwide. AIDS patients across the United States and throughout the world often cannot afford the medicine they need to help prolong and improve the quality of their lives. Unfortunately, congressional efforts to increase financial assistance for AIDS victims have been slowed by budgetary debates. Moreover, state governments, reeling from recessions and budget woes, have cut their AIDS drug assistance programs. As a result, many AIDS patients end up on state waiting lists to receive lifesaving treatment, and some die before ever receiving their first dose. The U.S. government must implement solutions, such as treating AIDS patients earlier when the costs of treatment are much lower. In addition, the nation must initiate a bulk drug purchasing system that would save billions of dollars and make AIDS drugs available to all in need.

Editor's Note: As of September 2005, 1400 individuals in eight states remain on waiting lists for HIV medications. This number includes those currently being served by the Presidential AIDS Initiative because there is no guarantee that their medications will continue to be provided once the $20 million temporary fix has *been exhausted. Both the House and Senate have allocated only $10 million to the 2006 federal budget. With one third of newly-diagnosed HIV positives qualifying for ADAPs, the program needs $313 million.*

President Bush's self-congratulatory AIDS speech staged at a strategically chosen Philadelphia black church . . . overflowed with all the obligatory visions of suffering, orphans, and tragedy mixed with glorious promises of funding, both global and domestic. Mainstream media and a majority of the U.S. public may have been duped, but AIDS activists, hardened by . . . recycled Reagan-era denial, remained unimpressed.

> ❝ *People with HIV/AIDS . . . have been forced onto 'waiting lists' to receive medicines they cannot live without.* ❞

Imbedded in Bush's speech was a promise of providing $20 million ("effective today") in emergency funding for drastically strained domestic programs that provide HIV medication to eligible individuals. After a spirited campaign effort rising in intensity [in 2004] consisting of phone calls, letter writing, visits to members of Congress, demonstrations, and support from a growing number of prestigious organizations, the president was forced to acknowledge the crisis. But, as with everything Bush, when the media hype fades, all that remains is secrecy, incompetence, more bureaucracy, and lives sacrificed for false glory.

As of July [2004], 1,629 people in 11 states were being refused treatment with lifesaving antiretroviral medicines in a funding priority gambit that placed more value on financing an unscrupulous war on terrorism than in assuring honorable management of a global pandemic here at home. As state and federal legislatures continue to be forced into slashing funding for medical treatment for the nation's most vulnerable and needy populations in order to balance strained budgets, people with HIV/AIDS (PWA) have been forced onto "waiting lists" to receive medicines they cannot live without. Left untreated, these individuals can expect to contract opportunistic infections and progression of their disease in a manner not unlike what was experienced during the disease's outbreak when no effective treatment existed.

Funding Fiascos

Medicaid programs are the largest public payer of HIV/AIDS care and medication, covering 55 percent of persons with AIDS and 90 percent of children with AIDS. Another major vehicle for dispensing HIV/AIDS medications to uninsured and under-insured individuals ineligible for Medicaid is the AIDS Drug Assistance Program (ADAP). It was created in 1987 as a means to help states purchase AZT, the only approved antiretroviral in existence at that time. When the Ryan White Comprehensive AIDS Resources Emergency (CARE) Act was enacted in 1990, ADAPs became incorporated under Title II of the Act. It is within these ADAPs that the present funding crisis exists.

Since 1990, the program has grown significantly, from $50 million in 1996 to almost $750 million in FY 2004. The CARE Act is a discretionary program as opposed to an entitlement and has to operate within fixed budgetary constraints. It does not receive automatic increases in funding based on need and must be refunded every year through a highly competitive appropriations process, causing yearly strain among PWA advocates and organizations reliant upon federal funding.

Bringing the HIV/AIDS issue to Capitol Hill was a bipartisan affair at the turn of the 21st century. Both Republican and Democratic legislators were quick to grasp the fiscal logic of treating HIV infection up front rather than paying for more serious, complicated, and expensive medical interventions that would result from untreated viruses left to replicate out of control. Since 2002, however, funding has consistently been inadequate. The budget passed for FY 2004 remains $180 million short, with only a $35 million increase for a total of $749 million. A $217 million increase for ADAP is needed for Fiscal Year 2005 (October 1, 2004–September 10, 2005).

State Budgets Are Tight

Along with inadequate funding on the federal level, ADAPs have been hard hit by state budgets reeling from economic recession and lowered tax revenues due to continued high unemployment and residual carryover from corporate investment scheme scandals. In FY 2002, states contributed 18 percent of the national ADAP budget. As employer-sponsored health insurance declines and the numbers of the uninsured increases, the outlook for finding ways to fill in the gaps at the state level has grown increasingly grim.

States have reacted by tightening eligibility requirements, capping enrollments, reducing drug formularies, and creating waiting lists. Patient Assistance Programs (PAPs) offered through pharmaceutical companies are an option, but the paperwork is time consuming for patients, doctors, and case managers. (With patients using three or more drugs in combination as standard treatment today, it is unlikely that all drugs needed by the individual will have been manufactured by the same pharmaceutical company, exacerbating the application process.) In a macabre Russian Roulette, PWAs are forced into a continuous holding pattern waiting for someone else to die, except that in today's world—at least in the U.S.—fewer people are dying. AIDS related deaths have declined by over 64 percent and utilization of ADAP has increased by 154 percent since 1996, when protease inhibitors were introduced as a new class of HIV medicine and highly active antiretroviral therapy (HAART) that utilized multi-drug combinations became the standard for HIV/AIDS treatment.

> *No one could imagine the terror of being told you would have to wait a month, a year, or more, to receive [AIDS] medications.*

On average 25 percent of the 40,000 persons who test HIV positive each year in the United States will be found to have progressed far enough along in their disease that they require immediate medication. Of those, 600 individuals per month are eligible to apply for medication access from ADAPs. Treatment regimens available today can control the virus' replication and forestall progression to the advanced diagnosis of AIDS, in some persons indefinitely.

AIDS is clinically defined as a patient who has experienced an opportunistic infection or whose CD4 count falls below 200. The United States Department of Health and Human Services (HHS) *Guidelines for the Use of Antiretroviral Agents in HIV-1-Infected Adults and Adolescents* recommends that antiretroviral treatment be offered to all patients with 350 or fewer CD4 cells or over 55,000 viral load. Persons on ADAP waiting lists have been clinically diagnosed as meeting these guidelines with prescriptions in hand to prove it; nevertheless federal and state governments have ignored HHS guidelines by denying them treatment.

Grassroots Action

At the 2001 Conference on Retroviruses and Opportunistic Infections (CROI) in Chicago, a handful of attendees brainstormed the idea of creating a new, broadly inclusive group of PWAs to address issues around new drug development, clinical trials and research, and treatment concerns such as side effects and adherence. Although some initially thought such a group might be redundant, others saw the need for "not an organization of organizations, but an organization of people," said Fred Schaich, a founding member of ATAC (AIDS Treatment Activist Coalition). After two meetings facilitated and hosted by the Center for AIDS in Houston, ATAC was born, modeled after a successful European organization.

> *It was reported that five people who had been on Kentucky's [AIDS medication] wait list had died.*

ATAC soon saw the dwindling commitment to fund treatment access programs—both federally and in states. Restrictions on eligibility for ADAP assistance and waiting lists had appeared. A conference call in 2002 that attracted 20 participants to discuss waiting lists for ADAP resulted in what became an ATAC working group called Save ADAP. At first it operated as an unstructured "virtual" organization with communication exclusively via email. As of July 2002, no activists had been dedicated to ADAP funding, but before year's end, 30 activists were roused to lobby for $160 million in Washington, DC for FY 2003. While they won only half of the requested amount, $80 million was considered a significant victory.

By mid-year 2003, the severity of the crisis took hold. Everyone who is HIV positive can remember the shock of that first test result and the second reality check—sometimes years later—of being told the disease had progressed to a point where commitment to a treatment regimen would now define the rest of your life. No one could imagine the terror of being told you would have to wait a month, a year, or more, to receive medications.

Waiting Lists and Politics

A July 31, 2003 letter addressed to President George W. Bush from ATAC quoted the National Alliance of State and Territorial AIDS Directors (NASTAD) who reported over 500 U.S. citizens on state ADAP waiting lists. One hundred eighty-seven professional and grassroots organizations, coalitions, foundations, and networks co-signed the letter, even attracting the attention of an organization in Nairobi, Kenya.

An amendment to the House Labor/Health and Human Services Appropriations bill offered by Senator Charles Schumer (D-NY) that would have added $241.8 million to the FY 2004 ADAP budget was defeated on a starkly partisan vote of 53 to 44. A compromise between House and Senate resulted in a final increase of $35 million being passed, still $180 million short of need.

In October 2003 it was reported that five people who had been on Kentucky's wait list had died. Two deaths had also occurred in West Virginia. Congress was flooded with over 2,200 personalized letters from HIV providers across the country responding to an extensive mailing campaign spearheaded by the American Academy of HIV Medicine (AAHIVM). NASTAD reported that, as of November 2003, the wait list had grown to nearly 700 people.

In December [2003], ATAC convened their first strategy summit at the Gay Men's Health Crisis offices in New York City. The coalition's Drug Development Committee was already established, working with the pharmaceutical industry and boasting representative liaisons to each company with approved drugs or drugs in clinical research. Save ADAP, in comparison, was relatively new and confronting an immediate crisis. Most of its members had never even met in person. The summit produced long-term strategy goals and established an effective communication structure.

In January [2004], save ADAP launched its "Message in an Empty Pill Bottle Campaign." Members of Congress and President George Bush received empty pill bottles with personalized labels and a message inside calling for support of a $180 million emergency supplement for ADAP. An ATAC-sponsored Washington, DC lobbying effort in February attracted clients of ADAPs, people on waiting lists and front-line workers representing 32 states. The 100 attendees helped create "the best grassroots event I've seen in 12 years," said Ryan Clary of Project Inform. Fully 40 percent of the nation's states were now affected in some way by budget restrictions. Members of Congress and President Bush received a letter signed by 450 organizations asking for $180 million emergency supplemental assistance for FY 2004.

The AIDS Lobby Gets Aggressive

AIDS activists again converged on Capitol Hill . . . for the annual AIDSWatch lobbying event organized by the National Association of People with AIDS (NAPWA). The three-day event was followed by a march, demonstration (that attracted nearly 1,000 participants), and civil disobedience on the steps of the Capitol during which 100 were arrested for unlawful assembly. . . .

[Soon] the Bush administration's grand plan for Medicare prescription drug coverage [came] under the threat of investigation looking for threats and bribery, hiding information from Congress, and misuse of taxpayer dollars to pay for TV advertising for the questionable drug card plan. At the same time, the nation's other medical insurance program, Medicaid, was being threatened with extreme spending cuts—this from a program that had already been eviscerated in varying degrees depending on the state. The Senate confronted an overall spending cut of 11 percent by 2009 in the Senate Budget Resolution. After receiving enormous grass-roots pressure, one week later the Senate voted to strip $11 billion in proposed Medicaid cuts from their FY 2004–05 budget resolution.

The House blueprint of this resolution called for imposing binding restrictive caps for domestic discretionary programs, including Ryan White and ADAP, and cuts in entitlement programs, especially Medicaid, the HIV Medicaid Workgroup said. In June, the Labor/HHS appropriations subcommittee was reported to be "under enormous pressure to reduce spending to offset the nation's mounting debt, recent tax cuts, and the escalating cost of war," according to NAPWA. A stridently partisan Congress left Washington for August recess leaving these and other serious issues unresolved. . . .

Behind such draconian squabbles, health of PWAs continues to be compromised. HIV positive people are ineligible for Medicaid until they become seriously ill and are determined to be clinically disabled with advanced stages of the disease. A Stanford University study found patients facing a "cruel choice: spend most of their savings on AIDS drugs until they are poor enough to qualify for Medicaid (HAART costs an average of $13,000 per year) or forgo the drugs and wait until they are sick enough to qualify for [Medicaid] under medical eligibility rules." The study found significantly lower death rates (66 percent less) in states with publicly insured AIDS patients given less-restrictive eligibility rules and more generous drug coverage.

Pharmaceutical Arrogance

In December 2003, the HIV/AIDS community became furious over Abbott Laboratories' announcement of a five-fold increase of ritonavir (Norvir®) from an average wholesale price of $130 a month to $650 a month for a 200mg daily dose. The drug had been best used to boost blood levels of other drugs in anti-HIV treatment combinations, after failing as a drug in larger doses. It was especially effective for those with few existing treatment options whose viruses had become resistant.

> *Many AIDS Directors remain unsure whether their states will receive funding or how the [AIDS drug] assistance will be managed.*

It was believed that Abbott's rationale was that the drug's use as a booster in combination with other drugs entitled it to raise the price to more closely match the prices of other protease inhibitors. Abbott had modified its patient assistance program to help individuals who needed Norvir and the price ADAPs pay for the drug had been frozen via previous negotiations through June 2005, but what would happen after was unclear. Plus, there was no deal for third-party insurers who would likely pass the cost on to patients' out-of-pocket expenses. ATAC Drug Development Committee co-chair Matt Sharp called it "one of the most blatant and heinous acts of pharmaceutical greed I have seen in my 15 years of AIDS activism."

AIDS Treatment News editor and Save ADAP member John S. James wrote in an email, the "case may be the biggest unexpected, overnight prescription-drug price increase for a life-threatening condition in all of human history" and cautioned that people "outside of AIDS" should not "dismiss the Norvir increase because it's for HIV and therefore doesn't apply to them." He said the "increase sets a precedent that can hurt almost anybody. And it moves us toward a world where the big advances of 21st century medicine will routinely be reserved for a rich or well-insured minority."

Generic medicine supplier Essential Inventions, Inc. filed a petition to request Secretary of Health and Human Services Tommy Thompson to allow for the licensing of the drug as a generic because the medicine had been discovered in the performance of federal research grants awarded by the National Institutes of Health. The Bayh-Dole Act, passed in 1980, gives the Secretary authority to "march-in" on each patent and license other producers to supply U.S. consumers when necessary to alleviate health needs or because the patent holder has failed to make the invention available on reasonable terms.

Illinois Attorney General Lisa Madigan, whose office is investigating Abbott, said, "Norvir is not like a hay fever medicine that people take to lessen symptoms to be more comfortable. It is a drug they take to survive." [Abbott has also suffered] an investigation by the Attorney General of New York, a California class action suit and a complaint filed with the Federal Trade Commission.

Fighting Abbott

Abbott Laboratories corporate offices were Fax-zapped. ACT UP/NY and ACT UP/Philadelphia members demonstrated at Abbott Laboratories' Whippany, New Jersey manufacturing facility on February 19 [2004], chanting, "Abbott Lies, We Die: Drop the Price of Norvir." Activists showered the facility with "blood money" and left a funeral wreath "in protest of deaths that will occur due to increasing pharmaceutical price-gouging.". . .

Abbott Laboratories publicly announced that chief executive Miles White's total pay had increased 20 percent from 2002, totaling $3.4 million. "The inflated compensation package comes just weeks after Abbott Lab's astounding announcement that they have increased the price of a key AIDS drug,

Norvir, by 400 percent—inducing anxiety and alarm in many cash-strapped HIV/AIDS patients," PRNewswire said.

Physicians supported boycotts of Abbott research, consultation fees, and some products, with the American Academy of HIV Medicine and the HIV Medicine Association registering complaints. The National Institutes of Health held hearings on allowing a generic version of Norvir under the Bayh-Dole Act and the Food and Drug Administration issued a warning to Abbott about its marketing literature, which touted Norvir's lowest price but for which the low dose offers no anti-HIV activity.

In July [2004] it was announced that an antitrust and restraint of trade lawsuit that had been filed against Abbott by the AIDS Healthcare Foundation (AHF)—the largest AIDS organization in the United States with clinics in the U.S., Central America, and Africa—had reached a settlement. But ADAP member and Project Inform founder Martin Delany was critical of the settlement and said that AHF had a "history of bargaining for its own interests to the exclusion of those in the community as a whole. . . . The net effect is that people are being forced, through the Norvir price increase, to fund AHF's programs—without their consent."

"The HIV/AIDS community will not cease its efforts to bring Abbott's injustice and disease profiteering to the center spotlight of what is fast becoming an inflammatory debate on the future of healthcare in the U.S.," said Thomas Gegeny, executive director of the Center for AIDS in Houston and ATAC member. "With any luck, the Norvir price hike will become a textbook example of what pharmaceutical companies should not do and may even push the envelope further toward reasonable price controls for lifesaving medications in the U.S."

Absorbing the Costs

ADAPs across the country, cash-strapped or not, have been reeling from the adjustment in accommodating the $20,000 a year wholesale price (three times as much as most other AIDS medicines) for the newest most expensive HIV drug on the market, Fuzeon (T-20). All previous antiretrovirals attack the virus after it enters T Cells. Fuzeon is first in a new class of drug called Fusion Inhibitors that target HIV on the outside before it enters T Cells and starts to replicate. The drug offers hope to patients whose virus has become resistant to all other approved drugs.

Because Fuzeon is protein-based, the body's digestive system breaks it down just as it does with food; therefore, it must be administered by subcutaneous injection. Fuzeon is first delivered to the doctor's office where the patient is instructed on how to self-inject. Thereafter, it is delivered directly to the patient's home in individual vials in powder form that has to be reconstituted under sterile procedures and allowed to sit for one hour prior to administering.

> *// Withholding medical treatment for people with AIDS is a form of control over a population whose only fault has been to be infected with a disease that incurred . . . political interference and moralistic stigma. //*

Medicaid does not pay for the time it takes doctors to teach patients how to inject a drug, requiring HIV doctors to absorb yet another cost. A majority of insurance companies define drugs that must be injected as a medical treatment instead of a prescription product, covering the drugs at the same rate as an office procedure. That may mean a high deductible and then a payment of 20 to 30 percent coinsurance, which for Fuzeon could cost $4,000 per year, *POZ* magazine says.

In a pattern that is being duplicated in other states, the *Wall Street Journal* (January 13, 2004) reported that North Carolina's ADAP ran out of money for new patients two months after enrolling its first Fuzeon patient. Buying Fuzeon for one patient created a wait list for three others whose virus was not resistant to less expensive HIV medicines.

Testing, Treatment, and Ethics

Visiting with researchers and clinicians at the University of Alabama at Birmingham in January [2004], HHS Secretary Thompson touted research that supports the need to treat HIV infections early because the cost of treatment is much lower and the outcomes better. Paramount to achieving that goal was the U.S. Food and Drug Administration approval in March 2004 of its OraQuick® Rapid HIV Antibody Test, the first test approved for use using oral fluid that produces results in 20 minutes. A jubilant Sen. Arlen Specter (R-PA) said it was a "giant step forward in combating the global AIDS crisis" by giving "new hope to those at risk of this dreaded disease." Sen. Specter's pronouncement was duplicitous since six months prior to this statement he had voted against the Schumer Amendment which, if passed, would have fully funded ADAP and truly guaranteed "new hope" for the global AIDS crisis.

The Center for Disease Control and Prevention has expressed alarm that an estimated 200,000 U.S. citizens are unaware they could be infected with HIV and supports an aggressive testing initiative to identify those individuals. With OraQuick® at the ready, those people could be lining up at the doors of ADAPS nationwide any time now. Yet few elected officials have seriously pondered the ethics of testing for HIV in the "medically indigent" when they may not be able to access life-saving drugs through cash-strapped ADAPS, said Gordon Nary, executive director of Medical Advocates for Social Justice (June 24, 2003).

"One might therefore question the morality of the national HIV testing outreach hype without the appropriate caveat" to explain there is no money to treat someone who tests positive. Nary suggests that in states where ADAP is closed or threatened with closure, "there is an implicit contract in HIV testing—if one agrees to be tested, then he or she will receive timely and appropriate treatment if the test is positive." Failure to do so invites a reoccurrence of the "pre-HAART resistance to HIV testing when many at risk for HIV did not want to be tested or know their status since the therapies available . . . offered minimal hope."

Writing in the *Journal of Timely and Appropriate Care of People with HIV Disease* (January 2004), J. Kevin Carmichael, MD advocates for establishing a minimum formulary that includes antiretroviral therapy, prophylaxis for opportunistic infections, and required immunizations. In the same journal, John Bartlett, MD, says some method of judging "severity of need" might be established.

Some Successes

In the wake of President Bush's Philadelphia speech, two successes have been reported, sans Bush. After New Mexico faced having to put patients on waiting lists in the near future, Senator Jeff Bingaman issued a press statement in July [2004] calling for support of a $217 million funding increase in 2005 for

ADAP and sent letters to the two top health care appropriators in the Senate. Soon after, Governor Bill Richardson directed the state secretary of health to explore options to reinstate $2.6 million into the HIV/AIDS budget and to reaffirm commitment to the Billy Griego AIDS Act, named for Sen. Phil Griego's brother who died of AIDS. New Mexico had been looking at implementing restrictions during FY 04.

Colorado's 315 people on its ADAP waiting list have been given a reprieve on life due to a nearly $3 million influx from the state's tobacco settlement, although it is described as a "one-time lift" to the program. Colorado has a "dismal record on providing life-saving drugs to uninsured people," the *Denver Post* reported (July 16, 2004), coming in second only to Alabama in the number of people "languishing" on its wait list.

Initial information provided by the Kaiser Family Foundation soon after the Bush bailout only provided information on three states—Alabama, Arkansas, and Iowa. Kaiser reported that Alabama, with 353 on their list, would receive about $3.52 million ensuring that everyone would be removed from the list. The state had carried a waiting list since 1999, making it the longest-running list in the country. Arkansas was mentioned as not receiving funds because no one was on the wait list on the "official" date when counts were made on June 21. However, state health officials and doctors testified that the state's appropriations were inadequate to meet state needs, and since then new people have been added to the list.

Iowa was slated to have their 16 people served by the emergency funding. Arkansas, Colorado, Indiana, Oklahoma, South Dakota, Utah, and Washington were anticipating "other cost-containment strategies," and Massachusetts, Minnesota, Missouri, Nebraska, New Hampshire, New Jersey, Oregon, South Carolina, and Texas anticipated new or additional restrictions during FY 04. With Colorado and New Mexico off the danger list at least for the near future, that leaves Alaska (with 7 people on lists), Idaho (13), Iowa (6), Kentucky (113), Montana (8), North Carolina (716), South Dakota (23), and West Virginia (35), quoting figures from June.

Silence and Inaction

Since the initial response from Kaiser on June 30, [2004] an eerie silence has prevailed. Bush's bailout has yet to see delivery of any medications and the process has been steeped in such secrecy that Beltway insiders, professionals, and respected advocates have all been locked out of the process. Many AIDS Directors remain unsure whether their states will receive funding or how the assistance will be managed.

Lei Chou of the AIDS Treatment Data Network, an organization that monitors ADAP data, says their model had predicted the emergency 18 months ago. "Whether or not they get the care they need will be more of a matter of the state they live in than anything else. It has become a kind of geographic lottery." If this scenario continues unchecked, the United States could begin to look like a third world continent, with states acting like individual countries and people engaging in migrations to states with the best AIDS programs. In fact, it has already been happening.

> *Doling out [AIDS] medicines piecemeal . . . looks a lot like willful and intentional genocide.*

Michelle Rachel England, MSW [Master of Social Work], social worker for the South Dakota Ryan White CARE Program, expressed such a sentiment in her press statement for a press conference that was held in conjunction with the Save ADAP legislative visits. Working with two individuals from different African countries living in South Dakota for a time, she said, was an "eye opener." When they returned to their countries of Ethiopia and Cameroon, both were able to access medicines more readily in Africa than in South Dakota. South Dakota is the only state that still does not pay for protease inhibitors, the one breakthrough class of HIV medicine that transformed the disease's treatment options in 1996 and has become a standard of care protocol ever since.

To see how irresponsible fiscal management and disregard for a state's most poor, needy, and sick plays out, just look at Oregon. Once one of the best places for people with HIV/AIDS to live, it became one of the worst in less than a year. After making drastic cuts in its Medicaid program, hundreds of people rushed to ADAP, which then responded by restricting eligibility, cutting the formulary and instituting co-pays, forcing clients to choose between rent, food, utilities, or medications.

Sane Solutions

One option that would provide access to antiretroviral medicines before PWAs become seriously ill is the Early Treatment for HIV Act (ETHA). Modeled after the successful Breast and Cervical Cancer Prevention and Treatment Act of 2000, it would give states the option of readily amending their Medicaid eligibility requirements to include uninsured and underinsured, pre-disabled poor, and low-income people living with HIV. Treating HIV early, when it is more easily controlled, costs an average of $14,000 per year, compared to $34,000 per year if treatment waits until the patient has progressed to AIDS disability.

A report by the Institute of Medicine (IOM) goes further than ETHA in strongly advising creation of a new national program with uniform eligibility, standard of care and benefits; and in ending the vast disparity between state ADAP programs that in many cases do not even provide for all FDA approved antiretroviral medicines or medicines that treat and/or prevent various serious infections inherent to the disease. It was found that Medicaid is unsuitable to meet IOM's needs because of "statewide variability in eligibility levels and benefits and inadequate provider payments that encourage substandard care."

The report calls for the program to pay the same discounted prices for antiretrovirals as it does for the Veterans Administration and other federal agencies. Patients treated by HIV specialists for their first regimen show higher rates of success, significantly lowering the cost of their lifetime treatment. The recommendations suggest cost savings over 5 years of $7.35 billion dollars to the federal budget and $10.35 billion to states (in 2002 dollars). By changing funding from a discretionary program to an entitlement, the yearly appropriations process would be eliminated, allowing for more stability.

Yet another rational solution exists, one that embraces the elderly, as well as people with HIV/AIDS, heart disease, diabetes, cancer, hepatitis A, B or C, congenital deformities, and any other malady of human existence. Michigan Congressperson John Conyers has proposed the United States National Health Insurance Act (HR676) that would establish a new national health care insurance program by creating a single payer health care system using the already existing Medicare program and expanding and improving it to all residents. The bill's summary says it would "guarantee . . . the highest quality and cost effective health care services regardless of one's employment, income, or health care status." It also identifies the current system as an "inefficient and costly fragmented health care system" and says it would "reduce overall annual health care spending by over $50 billion in the first year" by using "rational bulk purchasing of medications."

It could be argued that withholding medical treatment for people with AIDS is a form of control over a population whose only fault has been to be infected with a disease that incurred the most political interference and moralistic stigma of any in modern times. While difficult to admit, the exacerbation of multiple attacks on many fronts—from stifling comprehensive reality-based prevention messages that do not stop infection rates in marginalized populations such as gays and people of color where the epidemic still runs rampant to doling out medicines piecemeal while transferring billions of taxpayer money to support a war machine—looks a lot like willful and intentional genocide. Residents of New Jersey who participated in the Save ADAP Capitol Hill visits experienced firsthand the indifference typical of some Republican staffers. There's a war going on, they were told, and sacrifices have to be made.

6

Distributing Untested Drugs Threatens AIDS Patients

Sally L. Satel

Sally Satel is a physician and a resident scholar at the American Enterprise Institute, a conservative think tank.

Programs that distribute untested AIDS drugs threaten the health of AIDS patients in the developing world. The World Health Organization (WHO), for example, has been racing to distribute generic AIDS drugs to millions of HIV-infected people in some African nations and other poor regions of the world. However, these drugs do not deliver the same level of medication as the patented form. The weak generic drug makes it easier for HIV to spread and mutate into a more deadly drug-resistant form. WHO is also distributing a drug containing three HIV drug compounds. Critics claim that these fixed dosed combinations are dangerous when treating a complex disease such as AIDS. In wealthy nations, for example, doctors customize doses and drug combinations based on a patient's other conditions to minimize side effects and drug interactions. The WHO should find safer strategies to fight the AIDS epidemic in the developing world.

The World Health Organization [WHO] is racing to get medication to millions of people infected with HIV/AIDS. The organization's "3 by 5 plan"—which aims to treat 3 million people, mostly Africans, by the end of 2005—is an ambitious one. But maybe WHO should slow down before it causes harm to those it seeks to aid.

A red flag went up . . . when WHO announced that two medications on its list of approved HIV drugs did not meet quality standards. The drugs were antiretrovirals made by Cipla, an Indian manufacturer whose major business is copying pharmaceuticals invented and patented by other companies, mainly in the United States.

Generic Drugs Are Not as Strong as the Original

The problem? The raw data from tests conducted by an independent company (hired by Cipla) to evaluate two of Cipla's HIV drugs—drugs that WHO endorsed—failed to prove that those drugs would deliver as much medication to a person's system as the gold-standard, patented form of the pills.

In the case of HIV/AIDS medications, low concentrations in blood and tissues make it harder to keep the virus from multiplying and creating mutant forms, some of which will no longer respond to medication. When these mutated forms multiply within an individual or are transmitted to another person, resistant strains spread and the disease becomes harder to contain.

> *The longer that patients are exposed to inadequate doses [of AIDS drugs], the greater the chance for drug-resistant HIV strains to develop.*

Since the two Cipla-made drugs were approved by WHO in 2002 and 2003, thousands of Africans have taken them. The longer that patients are exposed to inadequate doses, the greater the chance for drug-resistant HIV strains to develop.

To what extent has this already happened? Who will contact these individuals and tell them to discontinue the medications? And what medications will they take in place of these drugs?

How WHO will handle this problem is not the only question the organization faces. Some global health experts also worry that it is promoting a questionable treatment in the form of a pill called Triomune, also made by Cipla, as its first-line medication in the "3 by 5" initiative.

Triomune contains three standard HIV drug compounds (lamivudine, stavudine and nevirapine), each at a fixed dose and combined together in one pill. WHO officials say a combination pill is easier to distribute and more convenient for users. Many Western HIV/AIDS patients take up to 20 pills over the course of the day, so ease of administration is no small matter.

But there are potential problems. WHO does not test drugs, and Triomune has not been approved by the U.S. Food and Drug Administration because Cipla has not submitted it. This is especially puzzling in light of the FDA's recently announced intention to expedite approval of fixed-dose antiretrovirals made by foreign drug companies.

One-Size-Fits-All Approach Can Be Harmful

Many health experts are rightly skeptical of a one-size-fits-all approach to a complex disease that doctors in the West routinely treat with a flexible armament of drugs, adjusted to each patient according to that individual's needs.

Specific drugs are switched often or their dosage strengths adjusted depending on side effects, progress of the disease and other medical problems the patient suffers.

A doctor's freedom to custom-tailor a cocktail is essential so that the resulting medicine does not interact badly with other drugs or exacerbate a particular medical condition also suffered.

In rural Africa, where sophisticated medical care is lacking, a calculable percentage of patients will become very sick or even die from the nevirapine component of this three-in-one drug. Thus the dilemma: the need to balance drug-related deaths and illness from using Triomune against the numbers of people who would go untreated altogether if aid agencies adopted a flexible but more expensive strategy.

As attention turns to the International AIDS Conference in Bangkok . . . WHO must regain the world's confidence and not foist unproven drug therapies on the world's poor and sick.

7

Providing Generic Drugs Will Not Help AIDS Patients

Robert Goldberg

Robert Goldberg is a senior fellow at the National Center for Policy Analysis, a free-market think tank.

Generic AIDS drugs are not the solution to Africa's AIDS epidemic. Unfortunately, AIDS activists are encouraging African nations to ignore AIDS drug patent rights and produce cheap generics. Tragically, these activists are more concerned about reducing drug industry profits than they are about saving lives. AIDS drug patents need to be protected to maintain steady funding for new and improved drugs that will ultimately save more lives. Instead of placing all their hopes on generic AIDS drugs, African governments must adopt programs such as Uganda's. Since Uganda initiated a program that targets risky sexual behavior, HIV rates have been reduced by over 50 percent.

W hen pharmaceutical firms . . . dropped a lawsuit challenging a South African law that allowed the importation and manufacture of generic AIDS drugs, their decision was hailed by the media and activists, who saw it as a victory over giant drug companies out to squeeze profit from a public-health nightmare in Africa.

In fact, the settlement is a tragedy. It will do nothing to improve HIV care on a continent where 26 million people have died of AIDS since the 1980s and a further three million are diagnosed with the disease each year. Rather, because it is part of a strategy to impose price controls and limit patent protection on new biopharmaceuticals developed in the U.S., the settlement will help ensure that this current generation of AIDS drugs is the only one we have for a long time to come.

Drugs and the Spread of AIDS in Africa

AIDS has spread in Africa not because drugs are expensive, but because most African nations have ignored the disease. Uganda, an exception, began a program of prevention and drug treatment to stop mother-infant HIV transmission in 1986. The incidence of AIDS there has decreased from 30% of the population in 1986 to about 14.5% in 1999.

It's a delusion to think that making antiviral drugs cheap, or free, will make millions healthier. Free food is available yet children around the world are dying faster from hunger than they are from AIDS. Free and highly effective tuberculosis and malaria drugs in Russia and Africa have done little to stop the spread of a disease that claims two million lives a year.

> *AIDS has spread in Africa not because drugs are expensive, but because most African nations have ignored the disease.*

In truth, AIDS drugs have been largely free in several African countries for some time, but have few takers. Pharmaceutical-firm donation programs currently have just four countries participating because of a lack of health-care infrastructure—including trained medical staff—and interest. Nor do patents pose barriers. HIV drugs made by Bristol-Myers Squibb, such as Zerit and Videx, had no patent in many African markets. Generic companies could have stepped in years ago; none did, because there is no demand.

Charitable groups have shamelessly joined in the calls for generic drugs, even though they know cost isn't the problem. When *Medicins Sans Frontieres* (Doctors Without Borders)—the physicians group that garnered a Nobel Peace Prize because of its reputed dedication to the medically needy—was offered the triple combination of antiviral drugs at $350 a year (compared to the U.S. price of $10,000) to serve HIV patients in Africa, it balked. The group has been behind every media campaign to limit drug prices and patents. But when faced with virtual freebies, it admitted it could only treat a grand total of 2,000 people in 10 countries.

Their response is but a glimmer of what is in store for HIV-infected South Africa as a result of this misguided approach. In 1997, South Africa passed a law that allowed it to ignore patents and import generic versions of drugs. Now, with the assistance of AIDS groups, it is seeking to buy or make generic AIDS drugs in violation of international treaties.

South Africa's Dilemma with Patent Rights

Bristol-Myers Squibb, to its credit, called the South African bluff: It . . . relinquished any patent rights in the country. Not that it matters: The South African government never once put in a bid for the company's HIV drugs or asked a generic company to copy them. In fact, minutes after leading drug makers called off their suit . . . , South Africa's health minister announced the government wasn't sure it even wanted to use anti-retroviral drugs and had no immediate plans for obtaining them.

South Africa, of all the nations in Africa, has been the most indifferent and recalcitrant in the face of the AIDS epidemic. The country spends $279 million on all drugs, compared to a defense expenditure of $4.2 billion. It spends even less to get poor and uneducated patients to take the correct combination of pills at the right time. In rural areas, where most people lack running water, electricity and proper nutrition, let alone health care, it would be impossible anyway. In urban areas, about half of all medications are stolen from public hospitals and clinics and resold into European markets.

> *[AIDS] activists want other countries to adopt laws allowing governments to seize any patent for any drug.*

South Africa would be better off following the Ugandan model and combining prevention with a program of cutting childbirth transmission of AIDS by about 50% with AZT, an

AIDS drug now available for pennies a dose. As *The Economist* noted, "it is reluctant to do so, though, partly because of its deep-seated hostility to the drug companies."

Which is why South Africa has become ground zero in AIDS activism. AIDS activists and consumer groups in America regard the South African fight against drug companies as politically useful because it puts firms on the defensive. They view the country's law on patents as the model for how pharmaceutical firms should be regulated in the U.S. Activists want other countries to adopt laws allowing governments to seize any patent for any drug deemed essential to public health and farm it out to generic companies.

All of this keeps Africa from building up effective drug and prevention programs. Sadly, AIDS activists and consumer groups such as Public Citizen and Families USA are more interested in eliminating profits from the pharmaceutical industry than they are in eliminating AIDS.

The truth is that the ultimate solution to AIDS is prevention. African countries need better public health systems, as well as a vaccine. That vaccine will require an investment in research and development that only private companies can make.

The price and patents of new drugs pose no barriers in poor nations if richer ones get serious about helping. The International AIDS Vaccine Initiative is a public-private partnership established to develop and deliver an HIV vaccine to the Third World. As its founders acknowledge, it can't succeed without preserving patents and higher prices in the First World, as well as protecting patents and creating a guaranteed, though lower-priced, market in the Third World.

But if AIDS activists and consumer groups had their way, vaccine research would die. Rather than allowing prices to remain comparatively higher in the U.S. and Europe, consumer groups will continue to push for price controls and cheaper imports.

Patent Protection Leads to Drug Innovation

Price controls and the wanton destruction of intellectual property will do little to improve public health. But they will reduce innovation. The lag in HIV research and treatment will condemn the African continent to deeper darkness and death. And for that, the AIDS activists, their uncritical followers in the media, and their monstrous certainty about the evil of the drug companies will largely be to blame.

8

Scientists Must Develop an AIDS Vaccine

David Baltimore

David Baltimore is president of the California Institute of Technology. He was chairman of the AIDS Vaccine Research Committee of the National Institutes of Health from 1997 to 2002.

To develop an HIV/AIDS vaccine, strong leadership is needed from the government as well as the medical and academic community. Vaccine development is inherently a slow and arduous process because of the necessity to conduct clinical trials. Furthermore, the AIDS virus has proven to be complex, which has made vaccine development problematic. As a result, many professionals involved in the development of an AIDS vaccine have become frustrated and have lost the sense of urgency that is desperately needed. Government and medical leaders must provide consistent leadership to ensure that the vaccine development process proceeds as quickly as possible. AIDS is a serious global threat, and a successful vaccine is the only certain solution.

For . . . more than 20 years, AIDS has been progressing relentlessly and predictably while medical technology has been stymied in its effort to provide a fix. We do have effective drugs, but they treat the infection at great expense and with great difficulty. And we know what will do the job: a safe and effective vaccine. After all, vaccines stopped polio and hepatitis B. The difference is that those viruses are highly sensitive to antibody killing, so the vaccines needed only to induce anti-

David Baltimore, "Steering a Course to an AIDS Vaccine," *Science*, June 28, 2002. Copyright © 2002 by the American Association for the Advancement of Science. Reproduced by permission.

bodies. But HIV, the unquestionable cause of AIDS, has evolved to elude antibody killing, thwarting our attempts to induce a broadly protective antibody response, even in animals. A test of an antibody-based vaccine is being run by an optimistic company, but few experts give it much chance of success.

There Is Hope That a Vaccine Will Be Discovered

Are we powerless? No. A century of study of immunology and protein structure gives us hope that there are ways of designing immunogens that will work. So we examine each detail of the virus's structure, trying to find chinks in its armor where an antibody might penetrate. But the immunologists hold out a different hope: that there is a second type of immunity—the activity of killer T cells—that can clear some viral infections and help antibodies clear others. Maybe we could devise a way to use this arm of our immune systems against HIV. Over 10 years of research has been devoted to this hope, and great progress has been made. But we are still at an early stage; testing of the most extensively evaluated candidate vaccine was halted because it is not giving sufficient evidence of immunogenicity. . . .

> **//** We ought to make every effort to provide the leadership and vision to ensure that [HIV vaccine development] will proceed at the fastest possible pace. **//**

We have a pipeline of potential stimulants of T cell–based immunity feeding into early-stage testing. However, little has been evaluated in humans even for basic safety (Phase I trials). The most promising T cell stimulant is a DNA vaccine followed by a viral vector; it is still in an early phase of testing. Thus, should all go well, we might have a vaccine in 5 years, but things rarely go so well in this difficult business. Few will be surprised if it takes 10 years to get to a licenced vaccine. One big fear now is that we will be able to stimulate T cell immunity, but the virus will quickly elude it by changing its structure a bit. Already in monkeys and humans there is evidence of viral escape from T cell immunity. For reasons that still elude immunologists, even if you stimulate immunity with a complex immunogen, the T cells focus their response on just one simple peptide structure, making it easy for the virus to mutate to resistance. So the T cell route to immunity may yet be a very bumpy road.

Leadership Is Needed to Find a Vaccine

Are we appropriately organized to respond to this devastating epidemic? A plus is that the U.S. government is putting more money into AIDS research, and specifically into vaccine development, than the rest of the world combined. But the academic community, while taking the money, is still working on a business-as-usual basis. By contrast, the National Institutes of Health (NIH) itself has set up an integrated unit dedicated to making an HIV vaccine. It combines protein structure determination, immunology, vaccine candidate development, primate testing, and clinical assessment.

Leadership in the vaccine effort at the government level has been diffuse and invisible. . . . When Harold Varmus was NIH director, the effort had high-level patronage and constant visibility. There is now new NIH leadership, and we can only hope that the new director will understand that he can have no higher priority than to deal with the AIDS epidemic. It threatens world stability, it kills Americans, and it is the greatest threat to those who can least understand the need to take precautions against infection: the poor, the underserved, and the populations of underdeveloped countries.

[In July 2002] the biannual International AIDS Meeting will take place. There is unlikely to be any exciting news on the vaccine front, because progress is slow. It is important to realize that vaccine research is intrinsically slow because it takes a long time to know whether a trial has been successful. But we ought to make every effort to provide the leadership and vision to ensure that this inevitably protracted process will proceed at the fastest possible pace.

9

Reducing Mother-to-Child HIV Transmission Can Help Fight AIDS

Jesse Helms

Jesse Helms is a former Republican senator from North Carolina.

Every year over a half million babies are born with the AIDS virus. The transmission of AIDS from mother to child is the number one cause of death for children under ten worldwide. However, this tragedy can be avoided. Drugs and therapies can virtually eliminate mother-to-child HIV transmission. In addition to financial assistance, the United States must help developing nations create programs and train personnel so that millions of infant lives can be saved.

[E ach] year more than half a million babies in the developing world will contract from their mothers the virus that causes AIDS, despite the fact that drugs and therapies exist that could virtually eliminate mother-to-child transmission of the killer disease.

It is my intent to offer an amendment with Republican Sen. Bill Frist of Tennessee to the emergency supplemental appropriations bill to add $500 million—contingent on dollar-for-dollar contributions from the private sector—to the U.S. Agency for International Development's programs to fight the HIV/AIDS pandemic. The goal of this new money will be to make treatment available for every HIV-positive pregnant woman. As President Bush would say, we will leave no child behind.

There is no reason why we cannot eliminate, or nearly eliminate, mother-to-child transmission of HIV/AIDS—just as polio was virtually eliminated 40 years ago. Drugs and therapies are already provided to many in Africa and other afflicted areas. Only more resources are needed to expand this most humanitarian of projects.

Entire Generations Are Lost in AIDS

The stakes could not be higher. Already in many African nations, an entire generation has been lost to AIDS. Mother-to-child transmission of HIV could eliminate another. Although reliable numbers are hard to come by, experts believe that more than 2 million pregnant women in sub-Saharan Africa have HIV. Of these, nearly one-third will pass the virus on to their babies through labor, childbirth or breast-feeding, making mother-to-child transmission of AIDS the No. 1 killer of children under 10 in the world.

There will be obstacles to achieving universal availability of drugs and therapies. Many African nations lack the infrastructure and trained personnel to deliver health care on this scale. Some governments may not be cooperative.

My amendment will provide the administration with the flexibility to deliver the necessary assistance while addressing these obstacles. For instance, if the new Global Fund to Fight AIDS, Tuberculosis and Malaria is deemed the most efficient way to deliver assistance, then the president can transfer money there.

> **" There is no reason why we cannot eliminate . . . mother-to-child transmission of HIV/ AIDS. "**

The United Nations has already set an ambitious goal of reducing the portion of infants infected with HIV by 20 percent by 2005 and by 50 percent by 2010. We can accelerate these efforts, saving hundreds of thousands of lives, with a larger investment of public and private funds now. Private contributions, either financial or in kind—such as the donations of the drug nevirapine by the German pharmaceutical company Boehringer Ingelheim—are an essential part of a successful anti-AIDS strategy.

In addition, national commitment is absolutely essential. The government of Uganda can serve as an example. Through the leadership of Uganda's first lady, Janet Museveni, that country has cut in half its HIV infection rate. . . .

I [have] said publicly that I was ashamed that I had not done more concerning the world's AIDS pandemic. I told this to a conference organized by Samaritan's Purse, the finest humanitarian organization I know of. Indeed, it is their example of hope and caring for the world's most unfortunate that has inspired action by so many. Samaritan's Purse is led by Franklin Graham, son of Billy Graham—both of whom I count as dearest friends—but the organization was founded by the late Bob Pierce. Dr. Pierce's mission was to "Let my heart be broken with the things that break the heart of God." I know of no more heartbreaking tragedy in the world today than the loss of so many young people to a virus that could be stopped if we simply provided more resources.

Using Power for Good

Some may say that, despite the urgent humanitarian nature of the AIDS pandemic, this initiative is not consistent with some of my earlier positions. Indeed, I have always been an advocate of a very limited government, particularly as it concerns overseas commitments. Thomas Jefferson once wrote eloquently of a belief to which I still subscribe today: that "our wisdom will grow with our power, and teach us, that the less we use our power the greater it will be."

The United States has become, economically and militarily, the world's greatest power. I hope that we have also become the world's wisest power, and that our wisdom will show us how to use that power in the most judicious manner possible, as we have a responsibility to those on this earth to exercise great restraint.

But not all laws are of this earth. We also have a higher calling, and in the end our conscience is answerable to God. Perhaps, in my 81st year, I am too mindful of soon meeting Him, but I know that, like the Samaritan traveling from Jerusalem to Jericho, we cannot turn away when we see our fellow man in need.

10

African Governments Must Acknowledge the Role of the Military in the Spread of AIDS

Alex de Waal

Alex de Waal is founder and director of the London-based Justice Africa, a nonprofit organization dedicated to achieving peace and defending human rights in Africa.

The African military culture is in large part responsible for the spread of AIDS throughout Africa. The soldiers of war-torn Africa, who are away from home for long periods and given authority and power over villages, often abuse their power, engage in risky sexual behaviors, and become infected with the AIDS virus. African armies have HIV infection rates that are two to five times greater than the general population, and some are thought to have rates as high as 90 percent. As these armies move from village to village, they facilitate the spread of AIDS. African leaders must respond to this crisis.

Aids activists and policymakers have a taste for military metaphors. They speak of 'fighting' Aids, 'mobilising as if for war' and, more optimistically, 'vanquishing' the disease. Some diseases—smallpox and cholera are cases in point—are amenable to military-style campaigns. But sexually transmitted infections are not. Measures such as the incarceration of sex workers by the

US police during World War I haven't often been effective. Policing sex rarely works. In fact, it's simpler to wage a war than to 'fight' HIV. States are designed for war-making. They have emergency powers and mobilisation capacities, while their leaders adore taking a posture of stern command. Even liberation wars, fought against states, invoke stirring slogans, promises of Utopia, and nationalist sentiment.

> **Africa's leaders should see Aids as their number-one priority.**

Speaking of the need for 'war' on Aids alarms people, and they should be alarmed. In some African countries, national survival is indeed at stake. For a country with 20-35% HIV prevalence among the adult population—that is, all southern African countries—the lifetime chance of contracting the virus for a teenager today ranges up to 70%. Statistically, a 16-year-old in Botswana can expect two decades of adult life, just half of her or his parents'. About 28 million Africans are estimated to be living with HIV and Aids. Not only is this an incalculable human tragedy, the loss of human resources stands as the single greatest impediment to social and economic development, and a huge threat to stability and security.

Aids Should Be Africa's Top Priority

Wars demand exceptional measures and clear and courageous leadership. Africa's leaders should see Aids as their number-one priority, laying aside all other national plans while they focus on the disease. So far, with just a few exceptions (notably Botswana), this is just wishful thinking. The 'war' on Aids is being conducted in a business-as-usual manner. It's a series of incremental programmes run by health ministries and voluntary agencies, mostly worthy but lacking the levels of both funding and leadership that are warranted. In fact there's very little strategic coordination at all: ministries, aid agencies and donors make relatively short-term, narrowly focused decisions about what to do. All 'fronts' in this war are important, but some are more fashionable than others. Mother-to-child transmission of HIV has gained a lot of (deserved) attention. Soldiers, policemen and prison officers living with HIV and Aids have not. There is something to be said for allowing each of those involved to decide where and how to expend their energies. It makes for innovation and voluntarism. That's how the deregulated market in aid to Africa operates. It is not, typically, how wars are fought and won.

The war metaphor is also misleading. War is a realisation of militaristic and, characteristically, masculine values, including hierarchy, command and obedience. In wartime, these values also permeate the personal and sexual lives of citizens. 'Fighting' Aids demands a rather different kind of 'war': a patient, frank engagement with some of the most intimate and deeply held beliefs and practices of communities and individuals. In this 'combat', governments and institutions should surrender some of their power and instead listen to ordinary young women and men. And even more to the point, men should negotiate sex with women as equals.

Better Tracking Information Is Needed

Truth is also, of course, a casualty of war. Here we run into a major contradiction: the 'war' on Aids demands intelligence, especially good epidemiological data: who has the virus, how they got it and whether they're spreading it. It's a shocking fact that the first 20 years of the Aids pandemic has produced such rudimentary epidemiology of HIV. Billions of dollars have been spent searching for a cure, but comparatively minuscule amounts on the kind of public health data that are useful in changing behaviour to prevent transmission. And a survey of the epidemiology will turn up one huge chasm from which virtually no information has escaped: the military itself.

> *Armies have played an important role in the Aids epidemic in Africa.*

This black hole is disturbing. A compilation of anecdotes and snatches of data suggests that armies have played an important role in the Aids epidemic in Africa. Right at the beginning of the pandemic, the pattern of Aids in Uganda in the mid-1980s reproduced rather precisely the progress of the Tanzanian army that invaded the country in 1979. This army had earlier been encamped on the western shores of Lake Victoria, the very location where many of the earliest cases of Aids were retrospectively diagnosed. What better vector to transform an isolated cluster of HIV cases into an epidemic than an army of young men, regularly paid, posted far away from home?

Sexual Violence Is Rarely Reported

Sexual violence is a statistical no man's-land. Indisputably, the reported cases of rape are a tiny fraction of the real number. Most likely, even fewer rapes are reported when the rapist wears a uniform. Rape by soldiers and policemen has only rarely become a public scandal. An exceptional case was the shockingly high level of sexual violence against Somali refugees in Kenya ten years ago. While most of it was perpetrated by criminal gangs known as *shifta*, a substantial number of rapes were carried out by the soldiers and policemen who were supposed to be protecting the refugees. Exposure by human rights organisations and a special programme by the UN High Commissioner for Refugees to protect women from rape helped overcome the problem. But, in the meantime, how many women became infected with HIV?

> **A big part of the blame for Africa's Aids epidemic must fall on wars, soldiers and cultures of militarisation.**

Rape has been documented as a weapon of war in a number of countries. There are stories of 'special' units of HIV-positive militiamen systematically raping Tutsi women during the Rwandese genocide of 1994. Mass rape has been perpetrated on women and girls captured by the Sudanese army in operations to burn villages and relocate their inhabitants to what they call 'peace camps'.

It is probable that most soldiers' sexual encounters are consensual. But that does not make the woman an equal 'partner'—the very word conceals the hierarchy inherent in most soldiers' sexual encounters. Army garrisons are typically surrounded by bars and brothels. Soldiers are paid well and regularly by the standards of rural Africa, where impoverished young women may be obliged to resort to 'survival sex': selling their bodies for the necessities of life. Officers' macho culture encourages multiple sexual 'conquests', and their status and pay make them attractive to young women seeking favours and security. The risk-embracing nature of military life makes a mockery of safe-sex messages. Why use a condom tonight when you may go into combat tomorrow?

HIV Infection Is High Among African Militaries

The UN agency responsible for coordinating Aids information and programming, UNAids, coyly remarks that HIV levels among African militaries are typically two to five times greater than in the general population. There are anecdotes of army units being tested and coming up with HIV-positivity rates of 50%, 70% or even 90%. A consistent anecdote is that HIV rates increase with rank and that they are higher among high-status units (especially air forces) than in the infantry. But we don't know much. The only published survey, conducted by the UNAids' Civil-Military Alliance, was carried out in 1995–96 and has not been repeated. Its data are now mostly a decade old. They don't give any reason for complacency: rates were typically 15–45%.

Governments Hide the Military Aids Problem

There are many reasons why governments want to keep Aids in the army secret. The reflex of the securitised states that dominate the continent is secrecy. Any indication that the officer corps, which is often the power base of the government itself, is riddled with Aids, might give solace to adversaries. They fear, it might tempt a neighbour to attack, or cause dissension or mutiny in the army itself. More immediately, the civilians surrounding army bases might become hostile to the garrisons in their midst. All African armies face the dilemma that if they were to acknowledge the scale of the problem, the costs for medication and care for soldiers living with HIV and Aids, and their families, would consume the entire defence budget and more.

Some African militaries have taken the threat very seriously. The first and most famous case is Uganda. Shortly after the guerrillas of the National Resistance Army had taken power in 1986, President Yoweri Museveni sent some soldiers to Cuba for training. He was quickly informed that a number (not disclosed) had tested HIV-positive. Museveni was newly in power and full of revolutionary energy, he had a very close personal bond to the young fighters who had won his war, and he also has a charismatic, frank and often humorous way of communicating. Museveni's campaign against Aids quickly became Africa's best-known success story. Not only has the country weathered the ravages of a disease that at one time was infecting more than 20% of the adult population, but it is the only case in Africa in which HIV levels have actually fallen substantially.

But there are reasons to question just how deep and long-lasting Uganda's success is. Recently, the chief of staff, General James Kazini, again remarked that Aids was a major problem in the Ugandan army. At war in Congo and Sudan, the army has lost its earlier discipline and dedication and is now better known for corruption. Despite constant military operations and attendant casualties, more than half the deaths in service are reported to be Aids-related. Soldiers who have been tested HIV-positive have also criticised the army for their treatment: medication has not been provided for them or their families and they have been victims of discrimination.

The Success in Ethiopia

Another, less well-known, case of the military containing Aids is Ethiopia. In 1996, discovering that the army had an infection rate of 6% (higher among senior officers), the chief of staff, General Tsadkan Gebretinsae designated fighting Aids as its number-one priority. Six years later, while Ethiopia's national HIV prevalence has risen to over 7% and the national Aids campaign has stagnated, the army still has a prevalence of just 6%. (In the interim it has recruited more than 250,000 men for a war with Eritrea, fought that war and demobilised many of them.) The key to the army's success seems to be a legacy from its years as a revolutionary guerrilla force in the 1970s and '80s which endowed it with some quasi-democratic institutions such as the 'council of commanders'. This, uniquely, allowed the Ethiopian army to have an open internal debate and adopt a set of anti-Aids policies by consensus. But, ironically, the same secretiveness that has concealed high military HIV rates in other countries has also meant that the army's success is not well known even in Ethiopia, let alone more widely.

These successes are too few, but there are signs of progress elsewhere. Senegal is an exemplary case for civil-military cooperation. The Tanzanian army has an open and enlightened policy, considering Aids in the military as an employment issue in which workers' rights should be respected.

Privately, African military commanders are expressing their fears more than ever. The Pentagon has become concerned, at first because US security strategies for Africa rely heavily on African peacekeepers. But the scale and nature of the HIV/Aids crisis in armies is still hidden. Shining a light into this dark corner is long overdue.

A big part of the blame for Africa's Aids epidemic must fall on wars, soldiers and cultures of militarisation. Declaring 'war' on the virus risks deluding leaders, both in Africa and globally, that the pandemic can be 'defeated' by further militarisation. Certainly, the campaign against HIV/Aids needs more resources and stronger leadership. But it will succeed if its 'weapons' are civilian and feminised, including gender equity, truly consensual sex, and frankness about all aspects of sexual behaviour. As Albert Camus remarked through Dr Rieux in the closing pages of *La Peste:* 'It's not a matter of heroism, it's a matter of honesty. It's an idea that may seem laughable, but the only way of fighting the plague is honesty.'

11

America Should Help Combat AIDS in Africa

Salih Booker

Salih Booker is the executive director of the Washington, D.C.–based Africa Action, the oldest advocacy organization on African affairs in the United States.

The AIDS epidemic in Africa poses a serious threat. Reversing the pandemic should thus be a top priority for the United States. Despite its vast wealth, however, the United States contributes only a small percentage of its foreign aid dollars to defeat AIDS in Africa. As a world leader, the United States should reverse this trend and divert some of the billions it spends on the war in Iraq to fight AIDS in Africa. In addition, U.S. trade representatives should promote policies that help rather than hinder efforts by African nations to fight AIDS. Rather than protect pharmaceutical companies, for example, the United States should make inexpensive AIDS drugs widely available. The United States should also support efforts to cancel Africa's foreign debts so that more money can be spent fighting AIDS.

At the end of 2002, President George W. Bush had a choice to make: go to Africa or prepare to go to war.

In December, while trying to distance itself from racist remarks made by then-Senate Majority Leader, Trent Lott (R-Miss.), the White House cited the planned trip to Africa as evidence of the president's and Republicans' concern for Black issues. But as soon as Lott stepped down from his leadership post, Bush canceled the week-long tour scheduled for January 2003 for reasons described only as unnamed "domestic and international considerations."

Bush's Africa trip would have been his first official visit to the continent and was to include stops in Senegal, Nigeria, Kenya, South Africa and Mauritius. The White House said the president planned to visit Africa to "continue building America's partnership with the continent and to share firsthand with African leaders his commitment to working on issues ranging from the war on terrorism to economic development."

The cancellation barely rated coverage by mainstream media. It seemed to accept that Washington had "more important" matters on its mind, namely plotting the invasion of Iraq.

Two months later, the White House found itself in the awkward position of trying to gain the support of the three African non-permanent members of the United Nations Security Council—Guinea, Cameroon and Angola—for its war plans.

> *The discerning observer can easily see that Africa should actually be a top priority for U.S. policymakers.*

Traditionally ignored by Washington, African countries are increasingly significant international players. The West African country of Guinea held the presidency of the security council during the fateful month of March [2003]. But despite the Bush administration's entreaties, the African members resisted the pressure to support the American war resolution and it was withdrawn.

For Africa, the importance of race as a determinant of U.S. foreign policy cannot be denied. It represents the initial barrier to an accurate understanding of U.S. interests in Africa. American society, which for most of its history has refused to value its own people of African descent, has also devalued an entire continent from which Africans were stolen and enslaved. Several hundred years of creating a national mind-set thus oriented are not undone in a few decades or by a few presidential trips.

But the discerning observer can easily see that Africa should actually be a top priority for U.S. policymakers if America is to focus on the most crucial global issues. Today's most urgent international threats, from the HIV/AIDS pandemic to extreme poverty, from environmental degradation to international terrorism, have their most immediate and devastating consequences in Africa. These challenges must be addressed in Africa, in partnership with Africans, if they are to be kept from overwhelming the world.

Facing the Challenge

The unprecedented challenges facing Africa and the United States are emblematic of the state of the world. The U.S. is the richest country in human history, while Africa contains the majority of the world's poorest countries. America's prosperity and Africa's impoverishment are historically linked.

The United States is now the sole superpower in the world. It has unmatched military and economic might. The U.S. faces the challenge of determining how to use its power not only to safeguard its own future security and prosperity, but also to promote the international stability and human security upon which America's own prospects depend.

Across the Atlantic, Africa is now the epicenter of the greatest catastrophe in recorded human history—the HIV/AIDS pandemic. Africa cannot overcome this challenge on its own, nor should it have to. But Africans must mobilize the international community to join their struggle to defeat this global public health crisis. And the AIDS crisis can be stemmed in Africa. But this would require not only attacking the disease, but also the poverty and structural inequalities that help fuel its spread.

> *The absence of U.S. leadership remains the greatest obstacle to a successful effort to defeat HIV/AIDS in Africa.*

The relationship of the United States to Africa graphically illustrates the central questions of the present era: How much inequality is the world prepared to accept, and at what cost? How should the United States address the historic injustices that are the cornerstones of contemporary western wealth and power, and that continue to define the pattern of global inequality? What are the obligations and motivations that determine America's international priorities? In short, what should be America's relationship to Africa?

Africa at Ground Zero

The HIV/AIDS pandemic and the wider health crisis that it represents threaten Africa's very survival. AIDS is also the greatest global threat to human security that exists today. This global fight will not be won unless there is a successful effort to respond to the crisis in Africa.

The statistics are alarming. Since its first appearance more than two decades ago, more than 18 million Africans have died of AIDS, out of 25 million AIDS deaths worldwide. Almost 30 million Africans are now living with HIV/AIDS, out of more than 40 million globally. Sub-Saharan Africa is home to 11 percent of the world's population, but more than 75 percent of the world's HIV/AIDS cases. More than 90 percent of the world's AIDS orphans (children who have lost one or both parents to AIDS) are African—12 million children, out of a global total of 13 million. In some southern African countries, up to one-third of the population is now living with HIV/AIDS.

> *The war on AIDS can be won, but the United States will have to increase funding significantly to help turn the tide.*

Health ministries in countries throughout Africa made significant gains in improving public health in the first decades after independence. Investments in health care by African governments in the 1960s and 1970s achieved improvements in key indicators such as life expectancy, which rose from an average of 44 years to more than 50 years in many countries. In Kenya, child mortality was reduced by almost 50 percent in the first two decades after independence.

But health indicators throughout Africa have fallen dramatically over the past two decades as a result of the HIV/AIDS crisis and other poverty-related diseases. Africa's health care systems have been unable to cope with the crisis primarily due to economic policies imposed on African countries by the World Bank and International Monetary Fund (IMF).

These policies—known as Structural Adjustment Programs—have forced cutbacks in public health funding and reduced access to basic services. The World Bank and IMF require countries to implement such programs as a condition for new loans as well as debt relief. They assume that reduced government expenditures and "free market" reforms will jump-start African economies. As a result, much of the social progress made in Africa's early post-independence years has been undone. Average life expectancy in Africa has fallen by 15 years in just the past two decades: in Zimbabwe from 65 to 39, in Botswana from 62 to 40, in Kenya from 66 to 48 and in Ethiopia from 51 to 41.

The social and economic effects of the current health crisis are devastating African countries. Schools are losing teachers faster than they can train new ones. The loss of millions of farmers is increasing food insecurity. These deaths are directly attributable to AIDS. Economic growth is declining, reversing all previous gains. The HIV/AIDS crisis is exacerbating Africa's underdevelopment and reinforcing the continent's vulnerability by increasing poverty and economic instability. Consequently, African economies are more negatively affected by external shocks (such as oil prices). Finally, AIDS is wiping out entire generations, thereby threatening the very future of some African countries.

This Disease Is Killing Mostly Black People

The absence of U.S. leadership remains the greatest obstacle to a successful effort to defeat HIV/AIDS in Africa and around the globe. While the United States has launched new initiatives to respond to AIDS in Africa, these remain wholly inadequate. President Bush has already reneged on the promises made to Africa in his State of the Union address in January [2001]. Declaring that America would provide $15 billion over 5 years, or $3 billion a year, to African efforts to fight AIDS and treat people living with the disease, the Bush administration, at this writing, has sought no new money for 2003 and only $450 million in new money for 2004. Projections for years further in the future are meaningless, both for people who will die without access to lifesaving drugs and for the U.S. Congress that can only appropriate funding for this year and next.

While this disease does not discriminate by race, or gender or geography, at present it is killing mostly Black people in

Africa, the Caribbean and increasingly, in the United States. As Peter Piot, executive director of the United Nations AIDS agency (UNAIDS), said just before the 13th World AIDS conference in South Africa in 2000. "If this would have happened in the Balkans, or in Eastern Europe, or in Mexico, with White people, the (Western world's) reaction would have been different."

The devastation caused by the pandemic in Africa is tolerated because of the perceived absence of U.S. interests there and the denigration of the value of African lives. If this were not the case, politicians would loudly acknowledge the obvious fact that the struggle against AIDS is more pressing than the war on terrorism.

Financing the Fight

The war on AIDS can be won, but the United States will have to increase funding significantly to help turn the tide. The Global Fund to Fight AIDS, Tuberculosis & Malaria, created in 2001 at the initiative of UN Secretary-General Kofi Annan, is a crucial new vehicle. The Fund needs at least $10 billion per year to finance an effective response to HIV/AIDS in the world's poorest countries, expanding both prevention programs and care for people living with AIDS. These funds could be provided easily by the United States and other wealthy countries, but the U.S. government has refused to make the necessary investment.

> *Funds [to support The Global Fund to Fight AIDS] could be provided easily by the United States.*

An appropriate annual U.S. contribution to the Global Fund would be $3.5 billion. This is based upon an "equitable contributions framework," where the 48 richest countries pay 90 percent of the total required (based upon each country's proportionate share of the global economy). Thus far, the U.S. has provided only $275 million, while pledging only another $200 million for this year. Italy has provided $108 million, Japan has contributed $80 million and Britain has donated $78 million. They've made comparable pledges for this year. Though the United States is the largest donor to the Fund, other nations are making greater contributions relative to the size of their economies.

Ideally, the private sector would contribute the remaining balance to realize the global target of $10 billion annually. This total pales in comparison to the hundreds of billions the U.S. is prepared to spend rebuilding Iraq.

Access Saves Lives

At present, about 1 percent of Africans living with HIV/AIDS have access to the life-saving drugs that have cut death rates so dramatically in the United States and other rich countries, as well as developing countries, such as Brazil, that have made them available. Ensuring access to essential medicines and care for all those living with HIV/AIDS is a global obligation.

Treatment is a basic right, and it is mandatory to defeat the HIV/AIDS pandemic. It is crucial to strengthening prevention efforts and to improving overall delivery of care and support. Treatment allows people living with HIV/AIDS to preserve their health, raise their children and continue to live productive lives. The availability of treatment is also an important incentive for HIV testing.

In recent years, the prohibitive cost of treatment, and the restrictive trade rules that have kept HIV/AIDS drugs out of reach for African nations, have come under challenge. U.S. policies have long sought to protect the profits of big pharmaceutical companies by restricting the ability of African nations to acquire affordable and generic medicines for their people using existing international trade provisions, such as compulsory licensing and parallel imports. Recent efforts by the U.S. trade representative at WTO [World Trade Organization] talks to restrict use of these provisions by poor countries were rejected by African officials.

A comprehensive approach to addressing Africa's HIV/AIDS pandemic must include measures to prevent the transmission of the disease from mothers to their babies. It must also respond to the AIDS orphan crisis by supporting care for these children and by providing AIDS treatment for their families.

Defeating HIV/AIDS in Africa will require a major investment in health care delivery systems and infrastructure. In particular, the United States should support efforts to improve the capacity of public health services in African countries. Washington should oppose the privatization of health care and the introduction of "user fees" for basic health care services. The imposition of these measures by the World Bank and IMF has been shown to decrease access to health care services for Africa's poor majority. Efforts to combat other infectious diseases such as malaria and tuberculosis, which cost millions of African lives each year, also warrant support.

Debt Holds Back African Efforts

Steps also must be taken to remove obstacles to African efforts to respond to the health crisis. The cancellation of sub-Saharan Africa's foreign debts, in many cases illegally incurred under despotic regimes, is crucial to stopping the diversion of resources from health care and social services. The servicing of these debts hinders the efforts of African governments to respond to the HIV/AIDS crisis and to provide adequate health care for their populations. Africa's burden of illegitimate and unpayable debt reveals a major failing of the current global economic system. It also represents a key source of global inequality.

Across Africa, debt repayments compete directly with spending on health care services. African governments are spending roughly $15 billion a year in debt service payments to rich country creditors and the international financial institutions, which is more than they are able to spend on health care or education for their citizens. In 2002, 10 African governments spent more on debt repayments than on health care and primary education combined. Meanwhile, 42 million school-age children in Africa are not enrolled in school. If Africa's debts were canceled, spending on education could be doubled.

Meanwhile, the debt that the U.S. and other rich countries owe Africa for centuries of injustice and exploitation remains outstanding.

The economic imbalance caused by Africa's massive debt is unsustainable and ultimately destabilizing, both morally and in terms of human security. Just as U.S. officials are now calling for the cancellation of Iraq's foreign debt, describing it as "illegitimate" because it was incurred during the reign of Saddam Hussein, so, too, should Africa's debt be written off.

Most of Africa's foreign debt is illegitimate in nature, having been incurred by unrepresentative and despotic regimes during the era of Cold War patronage. Many loans being repaid by African countries were made to Cold War dictators whom Africa's people did not choose and who used the money to repress them. Other loans being repaid by African countries were made to corrupt leaders who kept this money for themselves and added it to their own personal wealth.

> *The United States has a moral obligation, a historical responsibility and a national interest in helping to defeat the HIV/AIDS pandemic in Africa.*

In the Democratic Republic of Congo (DRC), formerly Zaire, dictator Mobutu Sese Seko received about half of all foreign aid that went to sub-Saharan Africa during much of the Cold War, even though it was known that this money was being diverted into his overseas bank accounts. In South Africa, the apartheid regime took out more than $18 billion in foreign loans in its final 15 years in power. The victims of the apartheid are now being forced to pay back loans that financed their repression.

African countries' debts have also swelled over time as a result of skyrocketing interest rates. Nigeria, for example, originally borrowed $5 billion from foreign governments and institutions. It has paid back $16 billion, but its debt still stands at $32 billion.

African countries owe a total of about $300 billion in foreign debt. As the All-Africa Conference of Churches, based in Nairobi, Kenya, has stated, "Every child in Africa is born with a financial burden which a lifetime's work cannot repay. This debt is a new form of slavery, as vicious as the slave trade."

The cancellation of Africa's illegitimate debt is essential to the continent's economic development. It is also crucial to African efforts to fight HIV/AIDS and to address poverty. While the United States is a relatively minor bilateral creditor of African countries, it is the single largest shareholder in the World Bank and the IMF, to whom most of Africa's debt is owed. As such, it holds major influence over the international response to Africa's debt crisis.

Do the Right Thing

The United States has a moral obligation, a historical responsibility and a national interest in helping to defeat the HIV/AIDS pandemic in Africa. As the wealthiest country of all time, it can afford to do much more. It can mobilize billions of dollars in domestic resources, which would leverage twice as much from other donors. It can also use its influence in the international financial institutions to cancel debts and dismantle the obstacles that impede African access to affordable medicines. America can still change the course of the global HIV/AIDS pandemic. This should be a top priority of the U.S. government.

12

AIDS Prevention Strategies Must Recognize Cultural Differences

Edward C. Green

Edward C. Green, a medical anthropologist, is a senior researcher at the Harvard Center for Population and Development Studies.

Activists developing strategies to combat AIDS in Africa must recognize the cultural differences between Africa and the West. Since Western AIDS activists believe that moralizing has no place in public health, AIDS programs in the sexually liberated West promote condom use and other safe-sex techniques rather than advise against risky sexual behavior. Africans, however, are still largely influenced by tradition and religion; thus programs that promote abstinence and fidelity have been more successful in African communities. Balanced programs that promote changes in sexual behavior combined with the use of safe-sex techniques will be more successful at reducing the spread of AIDS in Africa than would the safe-sex only programs used in developed nations.

While attending [an] international health conference, I sat in on a session on AIDS prevention. Out of the four scheduled presenters, only one, an American, showed up to

Edward C. Green, "Culture Clash and AIDS Prevention," *The Responsive Community,* Fall 2003. Copyright © 2003 by *The Responsive Community.* Reproduced by permission.

speak; the other three, all African, could not attend due to travel problems. The American speaker spoke about HIV transmission among gay men, using the word "homophobia" about a dozen times. The audience, mainly from Africa, Latin America, and the Caribbean, seemed unresponsive, and while there was at least 90 minutes left for a Q&A session, no one said a word. The situation seemed a bit awkward. The session moderator knew me, and perhaps because I was sitting near the front of the room, she asked me if I would like to open up a discussion about AIDS prevention. So I commented on the different patterns and dynamics of transmission between AIDS in America and Africa, and told the audience a little about Uganda's simple, low-cost ABC program, led by President Museveni: Abstain, Be faithful, or use Condoms if A and B are not practiced. The abstinence message urges youth to delay having sex until they were older, preferably married. There is a deliberate attempt to fight stigma and discrimination associated with AIDS, and to generate open and candid discussion about the epidemic everywhere, down to the village level. Information about AIDS and how to avoid it reached local communities through culturally appropriate means of communication involving local leaders, indigenous healers, drama, and song. There was AIDS education in the primary schools. Christian and Muslim faith-based organizations were involved from the beginning of the national response, and they are particularly adept at promoting abstinence and faithfulness. The government took concrete steps to empower women so that they could refuse unwanted sex.

> **"** *Africans . . . thought that promotion of fidelity and abstinence was exactly the right response to AIDS.* **"**

The result? Since the program's inception, Uganda has experienced an unparalleled two-thirds reduction in national HIV infection rates, and in 1989, the new infection rate began to decline. Western experts began showing up a few years later.

The audience was immediately full of questions: Why had they not heard more about these interventions? Why don't we involve religious groups and schoolteachers more in AIDS prevention? How can we prevent seduction of schoolgirls by older men? How can we get husbands to stop running around and then infecting their wives? Just as the audience had no comments about the presentation they had just heard, the American who had made the presentation had no comments about this new topic that so animated the audience.

A Clash of Cultures

This illustrates not only the very different types of epidemics found in two regions of the world and therefore the different responses needed to address them, but also a clash of cultures and values between the West and Africa. Africans and others in the audience thought that promotion of fidelity and abstinence was exactly the right response to AIDS, whereas this is usually thought by Westerners to constitute unwarranted infringement in people's personal lives. Some of my colleagues call this approach "missionary terrorism," designed to interfere with people's right to experience having multiple sexual partners. The American and indeed Western model of AIDS prevention is to leave sexual behavior alone, but reduce risk by promoting condoms and treating the curable STDs [sexually transmitted diseases] (since these facilitate transmission of HIV).

> *African cultures are still largely bound by tradition and religion, and . . . they have not undergone the general sexual revolution.*

How has the Western risk-reduction model fared in Africa? There is no evidence that mass promotion of condoms has paid off with a decline of HIV infection rates at the population level in Africa, according to a new UNAIDS [Joint United Nations Programme on HIV/AIDS] assessment of condom effectiveness. In fact, countries with the highest levels of condom availability (Zimbabwe, Botswana, South Africa, Kenya) also have some of the highest HIV prevalence rates in the world. Still unknown is the impact of the other relatively expensive AIDS prevention programs we now fund, namely widespread treatment of STDs or voluntary counseling and testing. We do know that these programs, along with condom social marketing, had not yet started in Uganda when infection rates began to decline. This does not mean they might not have contributed to the decline in HIV in later years. In fact, even though only 8 percent of Ugandan men and women were using condoms regularly by 2000, those who were using them were exactly the ones that needed them: sex workers and the relatively few men who still had multiple partners.

Exploring the History of AIDS Prevention

To understand why the major donors continue to pour millions of dollars into risk reduction while largely ignoring the evidence from Africa, it is useful to review some recent history. Western donor organizations and the groups they fund began implementing "behavior change communications" programs in the Third World in the mid-1980s, soon after American AIDS activists felt they had discovered how to defeat AIDS in San Francisco and New York. Of course, the very term "behavior change" suggests that outsiders know what is best for Africans, that Africans are misbehaving and need to *change* their behavior, and that outsiders will show them the way to behave. Yet now that we have comparative data, we know that African and American sexual behavior is not very different. There are subgroups of Africans and Americans who have a great many sexual partners, but *most people* in both populations do not.

When Americans designed interventions for Africans, the only prevention model available was the risk reduction model that had been designed in the United States for special high-risk groups. The model's premise was that we cannot change the behavior of gay men (or drug addicts), therefore the best we can do is reduce risk through condom promotion (and needle exchange for addicts). This model seemed to work in the 1980s, although infection rates are rising again among gay men in America. Nevertheless, since the mid-1980s, this model has been applied to populations where most of those infected are not in special high-risk groups but instead in the majority population. In short, we provided American solutions for Third World populations. Once the risk reduction model was launched in Africa and the developing world, it assumed a life of its own and became the unchallenged paradigm for global AIDS prevention.

The risk reduction approach also involves the promotion of "safer sex" practices such as mutual masturbation and oral sex, if not male-to-male sex, even though all these practices seem to be comparatively rare in Africa. Some Westerners see this as liberating Africans from outmoded and perhaps repressive sexual norms. What Americans and Europeans forgot when designing these approaches is that African cultures are still largely bound by tradition and religion, and that they have not undergone the general sexual revolution, and certainly not the gay-lesbian revolution, of the West. This should have been Anthropology 101.

In the minds of Western AIDS activists and public health professionals, no one should judge someone else's sexual behavior. This leads to "moralizing" about behavior, and which should not have any place in public health. Yet Ugandans who turned around their AIDS epidemic did not know they were supposed to remain value-neutral. In a BBC interview in August 2002, Museveni recounted how he talked about AIDS at every meeting with the public: "I would shout at them . . . you are going to die if you don't stop this [having multiple sexual partners]. You are going to die."

> *In the minds of Western AIDS activists and public health professionals, no one should judge someone else's sexual behavior.*

Forms of sexual behavior highly relevant to HIV transmission, such as rape, coercion, and seduction of minors, take us into the realm of morals or at least ethics, whatever our objections. Issues involving questions of right and wrong may well require an ethical or value-related answer. Ellen Goodman has wondered whether in the American transition from a more religious to a more secular society, we have somehow given ourselves a "moral lobotomy." She asks whether, due to our reluctance to being considered judgmental, ". . . are we disabled from making any judgment at all?" To avoid a fatal disease fueled by having multiple sex partners, good judgment dictates that people have fewer partners. Common sense should not be dismissed as moralizing.

Political and Economic Influence

Apart from Western values and biases, there are economic factors to consider. AIDS prevention has become a billion dollar industry. Under President Bush's global AIDS initiative, the U.S. will spend $15 billion, partially on prevention. It would be politically naive to expect that those who profit from the lucrative AIDS-prevention industry would not be inclined to protect their interests. Those who work in condom promotion and STD treatment, as well as the industries that supply these devices and drugs, do not want to lose market share, so to speak, to those few who have begun to talk about behavior. Put crudely, who makes a buck if Africans simply start being monogamous?

Financial interests aside, it is tempting to rely on quick technological fixes to complex problems involving human behavior. Condoms and STD drugs can be procured, promoted, and distributed, and all of this can be counted easily. With condoms and pills we have ready-made monitoring and evaluation measurement units, and these units are already familiar from decades of experience with family planning programs. USAID [United States Agency for International Development] often comments that it has a "comparative advantage" in the condom supply and promotion part of AIDS prevention. Yet other major donors could also make the same claim, leaving no one with a "comparative advantage" in promoting non-contraceptive, non-drug interventions focused on simple behavioral change. In fact, faith-based organizations have exactly this interest and capability, but they are usually excluded from donor-funded participation in AIDS prevention. Western experts, who often have backgrounds in AIDS activism and contraception, are predisposed to be suspicious about religious organizations. There is a long history of antagonism between family planning organizations and certain religious groups, notably the Roman Catholic Church, and more recently, the "religious right" in America. Some of my family planning colleagues fear that raising any question about condom effectiveness for AIDS prevention is evidence of a larger agenda to cut off funding for all contraception and to oppose the advancement of women's rights.

The Ideological Battle over AIDS Prevention

Part of the whole problem is precisely the "ever-increasing polarization between left and right." Some in the religious right *have* in fact attacked broader contraception and progressive social programs in the same breath as they have attacked the condom distribution (or "condom airlift") solution to AIDS. This has put liberals so much on the defensive that they will simply not listen to logical public health arguments on the need to address risky sexual behavior in a pandemic driven by risky sexual behavior. Partisans on the left and right are currently fighting over how the newly promised billions for AIDS prevention will be spent. The fight seems to have once again been reduced to condoms versus abstinence, forgetting that the lesson from Uganda is that a balanced, integrated approach that provides a range of behavioral options is what works best.

13

Talking Openly About Sex Can Help Fight AIDS

Hope Cristol

Hope Cristol is a freelance writer and contributor to The Futurist, *a publication dedicated to providing perspectives on the future in a variety of social, scientific, and economic subject areas.*

Talking openly about AIDS prevention will help control the spread of AIDS worldwide. In Brazil, for example, the government took the threat of AIDS very seriously. The nation instituted a program that included frank and open communication about risky sexual behavior and prevention methods. As a result, the spread of AIDS was controlled in a nation that was predicted to be devastated by the disease.

A IDS researchers in the 1990s expected the disease to devastate Brazil. Ten years later, the country's incredibly successful prevention efforts have proved those predictions wrong.

Brazil's government took the AIDS threat very seriously and took immediate action. Besides free condom distribution, the government initiated widespread education campaigns to get the message out in newspapers, on billboards, and even on the airwaves by having the biggest pop stars sing targeted songs on the radio.

Like Brazil, Uganda has also proved bleak AIDS predictions wrong. What sets these policy programs apart is their open communication about the disease. A frank, far-reaching dialogue about the nature of HIV/AIDS, modes of transmission, and ways of prevention is key, explains Kathryn Whetten, a Duke University health policy expert.

"In Uganda and Brazil, this discussion was started from the top-down, but it can come from the grassroots as well," says Whetten, director of Duke's Health Inequalities Program in the Center for Health Policy, Law, and Management. "When I look at other countries at great risk now, we may find that their governments will be less inclined to be so open."

Governments Need to Be Open About AIDS Prevention

Governments in AIDS-plagued Cambodia, Thailand, Nigeria, China, and India are conflicted about how to handle the disease. One reason is the shame associated with AIDS in these countries. Another reason is that strong religious beliefs—regardless of the religion—tend to prohibit open discussions about stopping the spread of the disease because the discussions involve sexuality and not just public health.

But it's not just Third World countries that would benefit from Brazil and Uganda's open-dialogue initiatives.

A Conservative U.S. Policy

The United States, too, announced new HIV prevention strategies [in 2003]. And like Brazil, the United States has stabilized the number of new HIV cases per year. Unlike Brazil, however, the United States is advocating sexual abstinence as its preferred strategy for prevention. Further, the U.S. awareness campaigns don't deal explicitly with drug use, anal sex, and prostitution.

"We are concerned about the conservative policies adopted by the [U.S.] government on safe sex and intravenous drug users," Paulo Teixeira, director of Brazil's National Coordinating Office for AIDS, told the Pacific News Service. Earlier [in 2003], the World Health Organization asked Teixeira to apply Brazil's strategies on a global scale.

Organizations to Contact

AIDS Vaccine Advocacy Coalition (AVAC)
101 West Twenty-third St. #2227, New York, NY 10011
(212) 367-1279
Web site: www.avac.org

Founded in 1995, the AIDS Vaccine Advocacy Coalition's mission is to speed the ethical development and global delivery of preventive HIV vaccines. It addresses ethical issues, critiques the work of industry and government, provides education and mobilization services, and speaks on behalf of affected communities.

American Foundation for AIDS Research (AmFAR)
120 Wall St., 13th Fl., New York, NY 10005-3908
(212) 806-1600 • fax: (212) 806-1601
Web site: www.amfar.org

AmFAR is a nonprofit organization dedicated to the support of HIV/AIDS research, AIDS prevention, treatment education, and the advocacy of AIDS-related public policy. AmFAR produces a variety of print publications, including monographs, newsletters, and journals.

Centers for Disease Control and Prevention (CDC)
1600 Clifton Rd., Atlanta, GA 30333
(404) 639-3311 • (800) 311-3435
Web site: www.cdc.gov

Founded in 1946 as a division of the U.S. Department of Health and Human Services to help control malaria, the CDC has remained at the forefront of public health efforts to prevent and control infectious and chronic diseases, injuries, workplace hazards, disabilities, and environmental health threats. The CDC publishes information about AIDS on its Web site.

Global AIDS Interfaith Alliance (GAIA)
Presidio of San Francisco
PO Box 29110, San Francisco, CA 94129-0110
(415) 461-7196 • fax: (415) 461-9681
Web site: www.thegaia.org

GAIA is a nonprofit organization comprised of top AIDS researchers and doctors, religious leaders, and African medical officials, most of whom are associated with religiously based clinics and hospitals. GAIA partners with religious organizations in resource-poor countries for community-based HIV prevention and care. It assists communities in developing locally initiated, planned, and led AIDS workshops and community-specific action plans.

Harvard AIDS Institute (HAI)
651 Huntington Ave., Boston, MA 02115
(617) 432-4400 • fax: (617) 432-4545
e-mail: info@eci.harvard.edu • Web site: www.hsph.harvard.edu

For almost two decades HAI has been dedicated to promoting research, education, and leadership to end the AIDS epidemic. It partners with organizations in Africa and other regions of the world to develop sustained education and training programs. The organization publishes a number of newsletters, books, and news releases that are available on its Web site.

Health Gap Coalition
511 E. Fifth St., #4, New York, NY 10009
(212) 674-9598 • fax: (212) 208-4533
Web site: www.healthgap.org

The Health Gap Coalition is an organization of U.S.-based AIDS and human rights activists, people living with HIV/AIDS, public health experts, fair trade advocates, and concerned individuals who campaign against policies of neglect and avarice that deny AIDS treatment to millions and fuel the spread of HIV. It campaigns to sustain AIDS-drug access for people with HIV/AIDS across the globe. The coalition publishes papers and reports on its Web site.

International AIDS Society (IAS)
Ch. de L'Avanchet 33, CH-1216 Cointrin, Geneva, Switzerland
+41-(0)227.100.800 • fax: +41-(0)227.100.899
e-mail: info@iasociety.org • Web site: www.iasociety.org

IAS is an independent, international association of HIV/AIDS professionals and contributes to the control and management of HIV infection and AIDS through advocacy, education, facilitation of networks, and scientific debate. It supports best practices in research, prevention, and care.

International AIDS Vaccine Initiative (IAVI)
110 William St., 27th Fl., New York, NY 10038-3901
(212) 847-1111 • fax: (212) 847-1112
Web site: www.iavi.org

IAVI is a global organization that promotes the search for a vaccine to prevent HIV infection and AIDS. Founded in 1996 and operational in twenty-three countries, IAVI and its partners research and develop potential vaccines. The organization believes that finding an effective vaccine should be a global priority and works to assure that a future vaccine will be accessible to all who need it. It publishes a number of publications, including the monthly newsletter the *IAVI Report*.

National AIDS Fund (NAF)
1030 Fifteenth St. NW, Suite 860, Washington, DC 20005
(202) 408-4848 • fax: (202) 408-1818
Web site: www.aidsfund.org

NAF seeks to eliminate HIV as a major health and social problem. Its members work in partnership with the public and private sectors to provide care and to prevent new infections in communities and in the workplace by means of advocacy, grants, research, and education. The fund publishes the monthly newsletter *News form the National AIDS Fund.*

National Association of People with AIDS (NAPWA)
8401 Colesville Rd., Suite 750, Silver Spring, MD 20910
(240) 247-0880 • fax: (240) 247-0574
Web site: www.napwa.org

Founded in 1983, the National Association of People with AIDS is a non-profit membership organization that advocates on behalf of all people living with HIV and AIDS in order to end the pandemic and the human suffering caused by HIV/AIDS. NAPWA is the oldest national AIDS organization in the United States and the oldest national network of people living with HIV/AIDS in the world. It periodically publishes the e-mail–based newsletter *Positive Voice Updates.*

UNAIDS
20 Avenue Appia, CH-1211 Geneva 27, Switzerland
+41.22.791.3666 • fax: +41.22.791.4187
Web site: www.unaids.org

UNAIDS is a joint UN program on HIV/AIDS created by six organizations. Its mission is to lead, strengthen, and support an expanded response to HIV and AIDS that includes preventing the transmission of HIV, providing care and support to those already living with the virus, reducing the vulnerability of individuals and communities to HIV, and alleviating the impact of the epidemic. UNAIDS has many publications and reports that cover a variety of subjects related to AIDS, which are available on its Web site.

World Health Organization (WHO)
525 Twenty-third St. NW, Washington, DC 20037
(202) 974-3000 • fax: (202) 974-3663
Web site: www.who.int

WHO is a UN agency whose objective is to attain the highest possible level of health for all peoples. Its Web site provides links to reports, news, and events on the topic of AIDS. WHO publishes several publications, including the *World Health Report.*

Bibliography

Books

Greg Behrman   *The Invisible People: How the U.S. Has Slept through the Global AIDS Pandemic, the Greatest Humanitarian Catastrophe of Our Time.* Northampton, MA: Free Press, 2004.

Catherine Campbell   *Letting Them Die: Why HIV/AIDS Prevention Programmes Fail.* Bloomington: Indiana University Press, 2003.

Jon Cohen   *Shots in the Dark.* New York: W.W. Norton, 2001.

Lawrence Gostin   *The AIDS Pandemic: Complacency, Injustice, and Unfulfilled Expectations.* Chapel Hill: University of North Carolina Press, 2004.

Edward C. Green   *Rethinking AIDS Prevention: Learning from Successes in Developing Countries.* Westport, CT: Praeger, 2003.

Emma Guest   *Children of AIDS: Africa's Orphan Crisis.* London: Pluto Press, 2003.

Jacob Levenson   *The Secret Epidemic: The Story of AIDS and Black America.* New York: Pantheon, 2004.

Raymond Smith, ed.   *Encyclopedia of AIDS.* New York: Penguin, 2001.

Gerald Stine   *AIDS Update 2005.* Boston: Benjamin Cummings, 2005.

Stephen Stratton   *The Encyclopedia of HIV and AIDS.* New York: Facts On File, 2003.

Patricia Thomas   *Big Shot: Passion, Politics, and the Struggle for an AIDS Vaccine.* New York: Public Affairs, 2001.

Flossie Wong-Staal   *AIDS Vaccine Research.* New York: Marcel Dekker,
and Robert C. Gallo   2002.

Periodicals

Carol Adelman   "Ensuring the Safety of HIV/AIDS Generics," *Lancet,* June 4, 2005.

Hilary Hurd Anyaso   "A Problem We Can No Longer Ignore," *Black Issues in Higher Education,* March 24, 2005.

Greg Behrman   "AIDS Fight Demands Serious Money and Serious Plan," *Los Angeles Times,* March 1, 2004.

Salih Booker	"To Help Africa Battle Aids, Write Off Its Debt," *Liberal Opinion Week,* June 3, 2002.
Business Week	"How to Get AIDS Drugs to Africa," April 23, 2001.
Richard Feachem	"The Real Enemy," *Washington Post,* January 20–26, 2003.
Lynda Fenton	"Preventing HIV/AIDS Through Poverty Reduction: The Only Sustainable Solution?" *Lancet,* September 25, 2004.
Laurie Garrett	"The Lessons of HIV/AIDS," *Foreign Affairs,* July/August 2005.
William Jasper	"Global AIDS Con Game," *New American,* June 2, 2003.
Bebe Loft and Mark Heywood	"Patents on Drugs: Manufacturing Scarcity or Advancing Health?" *Journal of Law, Medicine, and Ethics,* Winter 2002.
Sarah Lueck	"White House Gets Pressure on AIDS Plan," *Wall Street Journal,* March 25, 2004.
Rian Malan	"Africa Isn't Dying of AIDS," *Spectator,* December 13–20, 2003.
Jim Nelson	"The AIDS Deniers," *Gentleman's Quarterly,* September 2001.
Emily Oster	"Sexually Transmitted Infections, Sexual Behavior, and the HIV/AIDS Epidemic," *Quarterly Journal of Economics,* May 2005.
Howard Phillips	"AIDS in South Africa: A Historical Perspective," *Society,* May/June 2003.
Peter Piot	"In Poor Nations, a New Will to Fight AIDS," *New York Times,* July 2, 2002.
Thomas C. Quinn and Julie Overbaugh	"HIV/AIDS in Women: An Expanding Epidemic," *Science,* June 10, 2005.
Michael Specter	"The Vaccine," *New Yorker,"* February 3, 2003.
Brent Staples	"How Needle Exchange Programs Fight the AIDS Epidemic," *New York Times,* October 25, 2004.
Elizabeth Terzakis	"The Global AIDS Crisis," *International Socialist Review,* September/October 2002.

Index